Activated
Charcoal
for Health

Activated Charcoal

for Health

100 Amazing and Unexpected Uses for Activated Charcoal

Britt Brandon, CFNS, CPT

Adams Media
New York   London   Toronto   Sydney   New Delhi

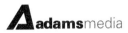

Adams Media
An Imprint of Simon & Schuster, Inc.
57 Littlefield Street
Avon, Massachusetts 02322

First Adams Media trade paperback edition OCTOBER 2017

ADAMS MEDIA and colophon are trademarks of Simon and Schuster.

For information about special discounts for bulk purchases, please contact Simon & Schuster Special Sales at 1-866-506-1949 or business@simonandschuster.com.

The Simon & Schuster Speakers Bureau can bring authors to your live event. For more information or to book an event contact the Simon & Schuster Speakers Bureau at 1-866-248-3049 or visit our website at www.simonspeakers.com.

Manufactured in the United States of America

10 9 8 7 6 5 4 3 2 1

Library of Congress Cataloging-in-Publication Data
Brandon, Britt, author.
Activated charcoal for health / Britt Brandon, CFNS, CPT.
Avon, Massachusetts: Adams Media, 2017.
Series: For health.
Includes index.
LCCN 2017021310 (print) | LCCN 2017031284 (ebook) | ISBN 9781507204672 (pb) |
ISBN 9781507204689 (ebook)
LCSH: Carbon, Activated--Therapeutic use. |
BISAC: HEALTH & FITNESS / Alternative Therapies. | HEALTH & FITNESS / Healing. |
HEALTH & FITNESS / Beauty & Grooming.
LCC RM666.C34 (ebook) | LCC RM666.C34 B73 2017 (print) | DDC 615.9/08--dc23
LC record available at https://lccn.loc.gov/2017021310

ISBN 978-1-5072-0467-2
ISBN 978-1-5072-0468-9 (ebook)

The various uses of activated charcoal as health aids are based on tradition, scientific theories, or limited research. They often have not been thoroughly tested in humans, and safety and effectiveness have not yet been proven in clinical trials. Some of the conditions for which activated charcoal can be used as a treatment or remedy are potentially serious and should be evaluated by a qualified healthcare provider.

CONTENTS

INTRODUCTION

If you discovered a product with healing powers that not only detoxified the blood and body and restored energy to the muscles and mind, but also provided anti-aging benefits such as fighting wrinkles, combatting cancerous growth in cells, and maintaining memory and cognitive functioning, would you be intrigued?

Join the millions of people around the world who have become interested in the positive effects that activated charcoal can have on overall health and the quality of daily life. This one unique ingredient has been developed into one hundred consumable and topical formulations that can help resolve health and beauty issues ranging from the reduction of high blood pressure and unhealthy cholesterol levels to the minimization of acne and wrinkles.

Natural gases give activated charcoal its highly porous surface, which helps it rid the body of toxins in a plethora of treatments, including shampoos that clarify hair, scrubs that cleanse skin, masks that clear pores, and soaks that detoxify the body. By integrating the applications presented in this book, you can transform your health, vitality, and beauty. The use of a small amount of activated charcoal can target specific health and beauty issues (which will be discussed in detail in this book), and a remarkable improvement in health can be seen in a short time.

Because holistic approaches to achieving better health have become more widely accepted by the general public in recent years, activated charcoal has now become one of the most popular and bestselling natural wellness supplements. A wide selection of activated charcoal manufacturers have tailored it for use in everything from meal preparation to beauty products.

By replacing the harsh additives and chemicals that are commonly used by food and drug manufacturers, activated charcoal can provide countless health benefits while ridding the body and brain of detrimental toxins that can lead to poor cognitive functioning, low energy levels, and pain.

On the following pages you will find one hundred benefits and ways to use this impressive ingredient in your daily routine to improve your health, beauty, and life in astonishing ways.

ACTIVATED CHARCOAL'S MANY HEALTH BENEFITS

What Is Activated Charcoal?

Activated charcoal, sometimes referred to as "activated carbon," is a form of carbon that has been specifically processed to have small pores. These pores help increase its absorption of elements and its ability to engage in chemical reactions. Because activated charcoal is manufactured for specific functions related to absorbing, expelling, or reacting to elements, it is sometimes referred to as "active" charcoal.

Manufacturers create activated charcoal from peat, coal, wood, petroleum, or coconut shells. Heating common charcoal with gases causes the charcoal to develop tiny internal spaces (its pores), giving it an astoundingly high degree of "microporosity." Even one gram of activated charcoal has an estimated surface area of 32,000 square feet! This activation process can be performed using either physical or chemical means, but both methods produce the same quality product.

The activated charcoal you find in stores and through distributors is derived from a variety of sources, but it's all created with the intent of ridding pollutants, contaminants, or chemicals from an environment. Activated charcoal can be used for a multitude of things, including removing air or water pollutants, making wine, purifying distilled alcohol, removing volatile organic compounds (VOCs) from products, and even cleansing the body of harmful elements. While activated charcoal has historically been used for medicinal or environmental cleansing purposes, it is now being included in a variety of beauty, health, and home uses that can all contribute to the improvement of your overall health and the quality of your daily life.

The History of Activated Charcoal

Charcoal has played a role in a variety of applications throughout history with the earliest recorded use dating back to 3750 B.C. It was utilized by the Egyptians and Sumerians in the manufacturing process of bronze, as well as a preservative. Even in construction projects along the River Nile, Egyptians used fire to char posts in order to prevent rot once they were implanted into the wet soil. After discovering the preservative powers of charcoal, the Egyptians began using the substance in their process of preserving the corpses of the dead. Once wrapped in cloth, the bodies of those who had passed would be buried under layers of sand and charcoal for preservation purposes. The Egyptians incorporated charcoal in their embalming processes as well.

In 450 B.C., the charring of wooden barrels was a common practice to prepare for the safe transport of potable water on long journeys at sea. In addition to water, a number of other foods and organic materials were transported using the charred carriers. This practice led to the fine-tuning of charcoal in water preservation and purification that has evolved into the effective filtration and processing procedures we use today.

The awareness that charcoal could be used for preservation or purification led to the medicinal uses that became popular during the times of Hippocrates and Pliny between 400 B.C. and A.D. 50. Once it was determined that charcoal had health-improving powers, the substance was used in the treatment of everything from epilepsy and severe anemia to vertigo and anthrax. Around A.D. 78, Pliny even wrote in *Natural History* (volume 36), "It is only when ignited and quenched that charcoal itself acquires its characteristic powers, and only when it seems to have perished that it becomes endowed with great virtue."

Following Pliny's documentation of charcoal as a medicinal staple, Claudius Galen, the most famous physician within the Roman Empire, researched and experimented with the substance, producing nearly 500 medical texts that detailed successful charcoal treatments for a wide range of diseases.

After the charcoal activation process was discovered and perfected between 1870 and 1920, reports of the successful medicinal use of activated charcoal became increasingly popular in published scientific journals around the world. Now regarded as a "safe and effective" application by the Food and Drug Administration (FDA), activated charcoal is commonly used in a wide variety of treatments in homes, hospitals, and clinics throughout the world. Available at a variety of locations and effective in countless applications, activated charcoal is taking the holistic healing community by storm.

How to Select and Store Your Charcoal

When activated charcoal is processed into powder, the original source can play a major role in its quality and intended use. Because it has such a wide variety of protective and preventative applications, such as gas purification, water purification, decaffeination, metal extraction, sewage treatment, medication, air filtration, etc., the consistency and porosity, or "grit," of the activated charcoal can vary just as widely. For example, in industrial, environmental, and agricultural uses, the most commonly preferred products have a larger hardness or abrasion number.

With organic, high quality varieties being easily accessible and low in cost, selecting the right activated charcoal for your favorite at-home applications is easier than ever. For beauty and health treatments, the activated charcoal should have a high density and low ash content. The fine forms of activated charcoal that should be used in personal applications are readily available in health stores and online, making the purchasing process very easy.

Once you purchase your activated charcoal powder, you should keep it in a dark area or cabinet, free of moisture and humidity. For most of the applications presented throughout this book, a simple teaspoon or tablespoon of charcoal is all that's needed. Combined with easy-to-find ingredients, activated charcoal treatments for health and beauty can be made simply and easily in your own home. In the rare chance that you are unable to find activated charcoal powder, there are countless locations and websites that offer activated charcoal in encapsulated or pressed pill form.

Special Benefits

Because activated charcoal has the ability to remove toxic chemical and organic compounds from air and water, it has been the center of countless studies performed to identify healing benefits within the body. Activated charcoal is readily used in cases of poisoning and drug and alcohol overdoses since it can rid the body of dangerous, harmful toxins. Additionally, activated charcoal has become a star ingredient in the treatment of blood disorders, cardiovascular conditions, digestive disruptions, and even brain and neurological conditions.

This odorless, tasteless, nontoxic powder is also an effective ingredient in a number of common external applications. With the ability to detoxify and naturally treat common skin conditions safely and effectively, activated charcoal can be used in the treatment of insect bites, athlete's foot, and acne, as well as in do-it-yourself makeup applications that safeguard your skin's health.

THE DARK (STAINING) SIDE OF ACTIVATED CHARCOAL

While activated charcoal can provide the body and mind with immense benefits when ingested or applied in topical applications, the processes involved in preparing these treatments can be quite messy if proper precautions are not in place. When you mix your activated charcoal be sure that you keep it contained in an area that will be easy to clean. Also because activated charcoal powder has a tendency to stain, wear only clothes that are able to be discarded if ruined. With these simple precautions in place, you can minimize the messiness of activated charcoal treatments simply and easily.

Safety Precautions

While activated charcoal is a nontoxic product, the safety precautions regarding its use should be acknowledged and understood before including charcoal in your everyday applications. With the ability to combat foreign and organic toxins, activated charcoal should not be consumed within two hours of ingesting medications as it will block their absorption. With excessive consumption, some studies have shown that diarrhea or constipation can result. Even though activated charcoal can be used in the treatment of digestive disorders, pregnant and breastfeeding women should always consult their physician before using the product in any ingested form. As with any product, the appearance of rashes, hives, or redness that might indicate an allergic reaction should always trigger discontinued use of the product. However, because activated charcoal is nontoxic and organic, irritations and reactions may be unique to a specific brand or manufacturer.

If you do choose to incorporate activated charcoal in your everyday life, it is always recommended that you consult your physician in order to determine if the product could possibly interfere with any medications, conditions, or illnesses you experience. Also, before you give activated charcoal to a child, please consult your pediatrician for advice and counsel.

PART 1

HEALTH

With pharmaceutical companies making billions of dollars annually preparing and providing the public with medications for almost every imaginable condition, illness, and disease, it's no surprise that the average American is bombarded with numerous advertisements and marketing strategies designed to promote over-the-counter and prescribed medications. The adverse effects of these medicinal treatments can sometimes aggravate current conditions, create new reactions, or even produce serious negative consequences that can lead to further disease or death.

In an effort to avoid complications, the holistic health community started delving into natural remedies for the treatment of common conditions and diseases. Just as certain forms of ginger, turmeric, aloe vera, and coconut oil can all contribute specific health benefits naturally, without the dangers of common synthetic medications, so too can activated charcoal. Activated charcoal has been shown to have unique properties that detoxify the body and support immunity against various ailments. It has been proven to fight heart disease and arthritis pain, as well as alleviate allergies and improve cognitive functions. With its ability to improve multiple physical and mental processes, activated charcoal can transform your health for the better!

1: COMBATS HEART DISEASE

Heart disease has become so prevalent among the American population that as of 2014, the Centers for Disease Control and Prevention (CDC) identified it as the leading cause of death among Americans. One out of every four deaths in the United States is due to this debilitating disease. Because heart disease includes a number of cardiovascular-related conditions, including strokes, heart attacks, and arterial conditions, the number of people who succumb to its life-altering consequences, or even death, has risen each and every year.

Thanks in part to research and in-depth studies focused on risk factors and preexisting conditions that contribute to the development of heart disease, physicians are now able to identify patients who are at risk and promote healthy changes to combat their chances of developing heart disease. While smoking, alcohol abuse, a sedentary lifestyle, and poor dietary habits contribute to the development of heart disease, genetics and preexisting conditions (such as diabetes and obesity) can also drastically increase the chances of a person developing heart disease.

Implementing activated charcoal in your day-to-day routine can reduce the incidence of heart attacks, strokes, and related conditions resulting from heart disease. Activated charcoal can provide the body with naturally detoxifying elements that can cleanse the bloodstream of impurities and improve the blood flow throughout the body and brain. It can also improve the circulation of naturally cleansed blood to minimize plaque build-up, negate the cholesterol within arteries, and optimize the delivery of purified oxygenated blood. By incorporating just 1 teaspoon of charcoal into your daily diet, whether in meals, smoothies, or even tinctures, you can alleviate the incidence of heart disease effectively and naturally.

CAUTIONS TO CONSIDER WITH ACTIVATED CHARCOAL AND MEDICATIONS

Activated charcoal's ability to trap toxins and impurities in the body and remove them naturally is impressive. There are cautionary conditions regarding activated charcoal that should be considered when the person who intends to consume activated charcoal is also on prescriptions or medications. With the ability to block the absorption of foreign formulations, activated charcoal may interfere with the body's ability to absorb or process medications, making it absolutely necessary to consult a physician regarding the use of activated charcoal when taking prescription or over-the-counter medcations.

2: FIGHTS KIDNEY DISEASE

According to the Centers for Disease Control and Prevention over 20 million Americans have some form of kidney disease. The kidneys are responsible for removing excessive creatinine (a waste product of muscle functioning) from the bloodstream. When the kidneys are overtasked with excessive creatinine levels, toxin overload, or even additives and unhealthy elements from a poor dietary regimen, the kidneys begin to fail. According to the National Kidney Foundation (NKF), this five-stage condition presents few symptoms until the progression has reached a serious level requiring medicinal or invasive treatments.

While diabetes is a major risk factor in the development of kidney disease, elevated blood pressure and blood sugar can also contribute to the onset and development of the disease. Because the condition is asymptomatic in the early stages, and because the disease progresses gradually over a period of years, the NKF recommends that at-risk populations be tested for abnormal creatinine levels in the blood stream regularly. (For example, African Americans are actually three times more likely to develop kidney disease.) Once creatinine levels have been evaluated, the patient's level of kidney function is rated as normal, mild, moderate, severe, or "end." If caught early enough, dietary and lifestyle changes can be implemented to return creatinine levels to normal.

Numerous scientific studies have followed patients diagnosed with kidney disease who have declined dialysis and opted instead for a treatment program focused on the daily consumption of 6 teaspoons of activated charcoal. Ever since these studies indicated resounding success in returning kidney function to normal levels, activated charcoal has been utilized in the treatment of kidney disease on a regular basis. Naturally healing the body and removing waste and toxic by-products from the bloodstream, this holistic substance is saving lives every day as a healing alternative to modern medicinal practices.

3: REDUCES HIGH CHOLESTEROL

While cholesterol is a natural aspect of metabolic processes and functioning, high levels of bad cholesterol (also known as LDL, or low-density lipoproteins) are associated with life-threatening strokes and pulmonary diseases, and even debilitating fatigue and energy loss. Because activated charcoal lowers the levels of total lipids, cholesterol, and triglycerides in the blood, it has a significant effect on minimizing bad cholesterol—equal to the effects of over-the-counter and pharmaceutical drugs that are prescribed to perform the same function.

While cholesterol has a bad reputation for being the main contributor to poor health, the body actually requires cholesterol in order to perform a variety of functions—the most important being the maintenance of cell membranes and structures. Cholesterol is also essential for making a number of critical hormones, such as cortisol, testosterone, and estrogen. Your body usually makes enough cholesterol on its own to preform these functions, but you can also get cholesterol from the foods you eat. Unfortunately, as is the case in many people's diets, you can take in an excess of cholesterol by making poor food choices. This overabundance can lead to a myriad of health problems, which is why it is important to rid your body of the unnecessary cholesterol.

When activated charcoal is introduced into the system, topically or orally, the main components of the substance are introduced directly into the bloodstream. With its clarifying and detoxifying capabilities, activated charcoal can eliminate unhealthy impurities in the blood (such as LDL cholesterol) and promote healthier blood content and blood flow. As the activated charcoal enables the removal of bad cholesterol, it also improves the functions of the heart, liver, and brain and decreases the risks of coronary artery disease.

4: IMPROVES GOOD CHOLESTEROL

"Good cholesterol" is a term used to refer to high-density lipoproteins (HDL) that help promote optimal functioning of the body's cells, organs, and systems. Cholesterol is required in a number of processes throughout the body, including the maintenance of cell membranes and walls; the processing of essential vitamins; the metabolism of fats, proteins, and carbohydrates; and the production of essential hormones.

While the body is able to utilize cholesterol obtained through foods, cholesterol is also created organically within the body. The body needs cholesterol to promote health and well-being, but when large amounts of cholesterol are consumed and fail to excrete from the body naturally, cholesterol deposits and complications can result.

By implementing a daily dose of activated charcoal in the diet, impurities within the blood stream that interfere with the natural processing of cholesterol can be removed. Activated charcoal absorbs unhealthy toxic wastes and impurities, keeping the the bloodstream clear of harmful elements that "block" the natural processing of cholesterol. This cleansing leads to improved cardiovascular function,

the ability to optimize good cholesterol, and a drastic boost to the natural systematic functions that provide energy, mental cognition, and metabolic processes.

With the addition of just 4–6 teaspoons of activated charcoal to the daily diet, the normal production of high-density lipoproteins can be restored, helping to improve everything from immune response to energy levels and mood. Activated charcoal provides a natural intervention that supports this area of health without the risk of catastrophic side effects that can result from pharmaceutical medicines.

ALLOW TIME BETWEEN YOUR MEDICATIONS

The only cautionary recommendation regarding the implementation of activated charcoal in the daily diet is to avoid consuming it within 2 hours of taking vitamins or prescribed medications. Due to activated charcoal's powerful ability to remove impurities from the bloodstream, it may interfere with the body's absorption of vitamins, minerals, and medicines.

5: BEATS BLOATING

Abdominal bloating is a condition in which your belly feels full and tight. Your belly might even look swollen in some cases. Bloating is almost always the result of consuming unhealthy drinks or poorly prepared foods that include excessive amounts of sodium, saturated fats, and preservatives. These overly processed foods contribute to the development of excessive gas, indigestion, and swelling of the abdomen. When the consumption of these unhealthy products combines with stress, anxiety, or upsetting emotional situations, the body can have a physical reaction that produces gases and initiate chemical reactions within the digestive system that can lead to bloating.

Even some healthy foods, such as the following, can produce physical reactions that lead to bloating:

1. Lentils
2. Beans
3. Cruciferous vegetables (broccoli, cauliflower, and brussels sprouts)
4. Artificial sweeteners
5. Dairy products
6. Whole grains

Consuming chewing gum, drinking through straws, and drinking carbonated beverages can also lead to excessive gas that builds up in the abdomen and results in bloating.

As a natural approach to combat bloating, activated charcoal can travel throughout the digestive system, cleansing the digestive tract and stomach of impurities and toxins that create excessive amounts of gas. The ingestion of activated charcoal in minimal amounts (1–3 teaspoons daily) dissolved in 1 cup of water one hour before or after meals can help alleviate the natural by-products that produce bloating without the complications of synthetic drugs.

THE IMPORTANCE OF HYDRATION

Everyone knows how important water is, but few realize how detrimental dehydration can be. Adversely affecting the entire body and mind, insufficient hydration can diminish the body's optimal processes and deplete the organs and cells of the water that's required for normal processing. With the recommended eight (8-ounce) glasses of water daily, anyone can relieve headaches, hunger, and low energy naturally while also improving the functions that the healthiest bodies enjoy!

6: MINIMIZES GAS

Flatulence is an embarrassing experience that can severely strain your everyday activities and responsibilities. While there are a number of over-the-counter and prescription medications that promise to deliver relief from excessive flatulence, these synthetic products often contain chemicals and additives that can produce harsh side effects and even complicate serious pre-existing conditions.

When bacteria in the colon ferment undigested food particles, gas can build up in the abdomen as a result and cause physical reactions such as burping, belching, and flatulence. The following foods have been determined to produce gaseousness:

1. Apples
2. Apricots
3. Artichokes
4. Asparagus
5. Bananas
6. Beans
7. Broccoli
8. Brussels sprouts
9. Cabbage
10. Cucumbers
11. Legumes
12. Melons
13. Onions
14. Peaches
15. Pears
16. Peas
17. Prunes
18. Radishes
19. Raw potatoes

An insufficient amount of an essential digestive enzyme, lactase, in the small intestine can result in food left undigested throughout the colon. If you find that gas is a common occurrence in your life, there is an all-natural solution that is safe, effective, and works immediately: activated charcoal.

Cleansing the gastrointestinal tract of impurities, activated charcoal not only helps rid the body of gas but also improves the functioning of the digestive system by removing the compounds that cause complications and disease. With a small 25–50 milligram dosage of activated charcoal in pressed pill or capsule form daily, any gas sufferer can find natural relief and resume a worry-free life without flatulence.

7: STOPS DIARRHEA

Diarrhea can be an annoying and uncomfortable illness that keeps you confined to your home within reach of a toilet, but it can also become a serious condition. The Centers for Disease Control and Prevention estimates that an average of 2,195 children around the world die every day as a result of the physical ramifications of diarrhea. That's more than the combined number of children who die from AIDS, malaria, and measles. If loose, watery stools last longer than three days, diarrhea can become a serious, life-threatening condition. The loss of electrolytes and the fluid imbalance that results from extended bouts of diarrhea can trigger the body's normal systematic functions to shut down.

Diarrhea sufferers who have diabetes, Crohn's disease, and ulcerative colitis can deal with even more complications caused by the depletion of essential vitamins and minerals and regularly produced enzymes. Indigestible foods, infections, bacteria, harmful organisms, excessive toxicity, and even stress and anxiety can all contribute to the development of diarrhea. While many over-the-counter medications promise to relieve the condition, the synthetic chemicals and additives can sometimes cause serious side effects or even further complicate the current diarrhea condition.

Using activated charcoal to resolve diarrhea causes toxins, bacteria, viruses, and microorganisms to be absorbed and removed from the body. Activated charcoal's electrostatic attraction to harmful chemicals and toxins helps the body resume normal bowel functioning quickly and easily without the harsh side effects of other medicinal therapies. Additionally, activated charcoal helps restore vitamin, mineral, and electrolyte levels back to normal.

THE IMPORTANCE OF HYDRATION DURING DIARRHEA

With the onset of diarrhea, the digestive system rids the body of bothersome bacteria, viruses, or microbes that are responsible for the upset. Unfortunately, along with this ridding is the extreme purging of the liquids and electrolytes on which the body's cells, organs, and systems heavily rely in order to function. In an effort to keep these essential components readily available, it is important to consume adequate amounts of water (at least eight to twelve (8-ounce) glasses of water per 24-hour period) during and after a bout of diarrhea.

8: REDUCES THE INCIDENCE OF INDIGESTION

The abdominal pain, burning sensation in the upper abdomen, heartburn, nausea, bloating, belching, flatulence, and vomiting that typically coincide with the onset of indigestion can be a major interference in normal day-to-day activities, leaving indigestion sufferers desperate for a solution.

While medicines may seem like a quick and easy option to rid oneself of this condition, the side effects, synthetic ingredients, and additives can be quite concerning. In an effort to naturally reduce the incidence of indigestion, homeopathic and naturalistic healing communities have utilized a combination of dietary and lifestyle changes in conjunction with activated charcoal, providing patients with astounding success.

Medical professionals and holistic healers have recommended that indigestion sufferers refrain from eating within three to four hours of bedtime, consume smaller meals more frequently throughout the day, avoid acidic and processed foods, opt for fresh fruits and vegetables, and exercise daily.

Following these recommendations may lead to relief for some indigestion sufferers, but it's important to note that the addition of activated charcoal has increased the success rate of curing indigestion immensely. Consuming a simple teaspoon of activated charcoal dissolved in 1 cup of water or taking activated charcoal in a pressed pill form can calm the enzymatic activities and chemical reactions that contribute to the development of indigestion. Activated charcoal can be used simply and easily, helping to alleviate and ultimately resolve indigestion completely without any side effects or chronic condition aggravation.

BEATING INDIGESTION BY BEATING STRESS

Whether it be a move, a divorce, or the birth of a baby, major changes and transitions in life can wreak havoc on the body and mind. Even if the change is a positive one, major shifts in daily routines, expectations, or work responsibilities can cause physical manifestations of stress like indigestion. Through adequate sleep, meditation, and exercise, the stress of any life situation can be minimized, and the incidence of indigestion can be resolved…naturally.

9: BEATS BAD BREATH

An estimated 99 percent of Americans (almost the entire population!) reportedly suffer from "morning breath." While the isolated morning bad breath can be quickly remedied with a simple brushing session and swish of mouthwash, a large percentage of people suffer with chronic bad breath, or "halitosis," throughout the day and find that it can't be resolved with readily available oral hygiene products.

Once thought to be predetermined by one's efficiency with regular oral hygiene applications, halitosis has been linked to a number of systematic dysfunctions throughout the body that contribute to the buildup of bacteria in the digestive system, bloodstream, and (of course) the mouth. By consuming activated charcoal, the physical conditions that contribute to chronic halitosis can be remedied naturally.

As activated charcoal is ingested, the toxin-absorbing powder cleanses the mouth of impurities that contribute to foul-smelling breath. Traveling through the digestive system, it improves the natural balance of essential nutrients, boosting the systematic functions of digestion and waste removal. All of these actions contribute to the resolution of halitosis, with the added benefit of overall health improvement. A simple teaspoon of activated charcoal powder can be combined with water to create a paste or mouthwash solution that can be swished around the mouth for 30–60 seconds and spit out to prevent the incidence of halitosis gradually over time.

THE NOT-SO-SWEET SIDE OF GUM

Whether the goal is to minimize bad breath, reduce common food cravings, or quit smoking, chewing gum can be quite handy. While seemingly harmless, convenient, and helpful, the artificial sweeteners and high sugar content in gum can have adverse effects on health. Whether manifested as dips and spikes in energy levels, nutritional deficiencies, or even dehydration, the consequences of excessive gum consumption can be catastrophic. By drinking water and teas, chewing on hydrating foods like celery and cucumber, and even napping, gum chewing habits can easily be replaced by healthier alternatives that simultaneously improve quality of life.

10: BATTLES BODY ODOR

A quick perusal of any personal care aisle at the local drugstore or grocery store makes the supply and demand for body odor relieving products quite apparent. By buying soaps, lotions, deodorants, and perfumes, countless Americans contribute to the multibillion-dollar industry that promises to deliver an artificial, sweet-smelling alternative to the body's natural, sometimes not-so-sweet, scent.

Body odor has many causes, including excessive sweating, stressful situations, poor dietary habits, neglectful hygiene practices, and even taking certain medications. Deodorizing products may seem safe because they're regularly used by a majority of the population, but several studies have determined that their use or overuse can actually cause the body to produce more foul-smelling bacteria and rid the body of healthy bacteria that would normally combat body odor. For example, in Belgium, a controlled clinical trial compared two groups: one that used deodorant and one that abstained from the use of deodorant for a period of eight weeks. The study determined that unpleasant body odor was more pungent and consistent in the group that used deodorizing products.

When activated charcoal is consumed and applied topically, the benefits not only include a reduction in the toxicity of the bloodstream and digestive system, but also the removal of unhealthy bacteria and microorganisms on the skin's surface that can contribute to the development of foul-smelling body odor. By consuming 1 teaspoon of activated charcoal dissolved in ½–1 cup of water daily and using activated charcoal–infused products (such as the soaps, soaks, and lotions listed in the Beauty section of this book), anyone can combat the natural incidence of body odor simply, easily, and naturally.

11: DISINFECTS WOUNDS

It is estimated that 6.5 million Americans suffer from chronic wound issues every year. Defined as "a wound that doesn't heal in an orderly set of stages and within a predictable amount of time," chronic wounds can take between three weeks and six months to heal. Those with chronic conditions that compromise the body's immune system and metabolic functions have the highest prevalence of chronic wounds, and also the longest wound recovery times.

While some wounds can be debilitating, most allow for a continuation of regular exercise that can help ensure adequate blood circulation for optimal delivery of white blood cells to the wound, speeding the healing process. In addition to exercise, a healthy diet consisting of nutrient-dense fruits, vegetables, healthy fats, and whole grains can guarantee that the body receives proper nutrition for wound healing, including essential vitamins and minerals that the body's organs and systems utilize for the very processes related to healing. By incorporating these two healthy habits into daily regimens, any wound-sufferer can naturally expedite and support the healing of a wound. As an added benefit, these habits also improve the immune system's functioning to better aid in the recovery from a wound and minimize the risk of infection. With all of the risks involved with wounds, the implementation of these lifestyle changes and the introduction of activated charcoal can safeguard overall health and well-being by speeding wound healing and minimizing infection at the site of the wound.

Ingested and topical forms of activated charcoal remove toxins from the body's skin surface as well as internal systems and also combat organic organisms that can prolong wound healing. A simple teaspoon of ingested activated charcoal dissolved in 1 cup of water can help restore the natural balance of the body's systems and specific organ functions. Soaps, salves, and soaks containing activated charcoal powder can topically extract toxins, allergens, and irritants from the wound to ensure the healthiest possible conditions and optimal healing times.

12: HELPS PREVENT HANGOVERS

After a night of drinking, the body's physical and mental processes can be seriously compromised with the onset of the dreaded hangover. Because there's no perfect formula to determine how much alcohol is "safe" to consume in order to avoid a hangover, any amount of alcohol can combine with a number of other factors, such as gender, age, weight, diet, lifestyle habits, and so on, to create the perfect scenario for the morning-after hangover.

Countless studies have been conducted to determine the causes of hangovers. The most widely accepted information outlines a hangover's causes as a severe drop in blood alcohol levels coupled with dehydration, increases in stomach acid production, loss of essential minerals and electrolytes, and dilation of blood vessels. The most common results of these physical conditions include:

1. Indigestion
2. Nausea
3. Vomiting
4. Headache
5. Body ache
6. Fatigue
7. Weakness
8. Shakiness
9. Increased sensitivity to light and sound
10. Inability to concentrate
11. Moodiness
12. Depression
13. Anxiety
14. Rapid heartbeat

In an effort to prevent the onset of hangovers, many people choose to proactively increase their nutrient consumption (vitamins and minerals), increase their water consumption, and get adequate rest. When these measures don't work and a hangover results, activated charcoal can help immensely.

With its ability to absorb toxins and chemicals that contribute to interferences with normal system functions throughout the brain and body, activated charcoal is able to help restore a natural balance following a night of excessive alcohol consumption. Used in hospitals and clinics around the world as the most common treatment for alcohol poisoning, a simple teaspoon serving of activated charcoal dissolved in 1 cup of water can help reverse the damage done the night before and minimize the physical and mental upsets of the dreaded hangover.

13: PROVIDES DIGESTIVE CLEANSING

There is a prevalence of toxins and harmful compounds in the environment, water supply, and food products that the body is exposed to on a regular basis. These toxic substances negate the natural functions of the body's organs and systems, making it imperative to minimize exposure to environmental and organic compounds and take proactive measures to purge the body of those that have been internalized already.

Even though the digestive system contains an astounding percentage of enzymes and metabolic processing components that help rid the body of toxins and maintain proper immunity, performing a digestive cleansing has been shown to relieve the body of harmful substances and restore a natural balance to organs, systems, and functions. One approach to digestive cleansing is the use of activated charcoal for detoxification and restoration of natural balance in enzymes, vitamins, minerals, and other organic compounds that are utilized by the body regularly.

The popularity of digestive cleansing products and services has skyrocketed in recent years. There are countless diets, juices, pills, potions, and tinctures that guarantee they are safe and effective. However, many of these programs and products contain synthetic ingredients and additives that can create serious health conditions that interfere with daily life or complicate current health conditions. Diarrhea, fatigue, nausea, vomiting, constipation, and even toxemia can all result from unhealthy approaches to digestive cleansing.

With a combination of 1 teaspoon of activated charcoal dissolved into 1 cup of water, along with a diet rich in fibrous fruits (like apples) and cruciferous vegetables (like broccoli), and an adequate intake of water, the digestive cleansing process can be performed naturally, without concern for harmful side effects and complications.

14: DETOXIFIES YOUR SYSTEM

Detoxification has become a widely used term to describe every program, product, and service that is intended to draw out impurities from the bloodstream, organs, and other elements of the brain and body, but few of these idealistic options deliver true detoxification. When the body is exposed to toxic elements, the buildup of foreign materials and organic compounds can be hazardous to health. Because the buildup of toxins can complicate the natural systematic processes of the body, it is imperative to maintain a toxin-free, homeostatic environment in the brain and body in order to live a long life free of illness and disease.

By avoiding unhealthy dietary and lifestyle habits such as smoking, consuming fatty, processed foods, and ingesting excessive amounts of alcohol or drugs, you can start preventing toxicity in the body. Incorporating activated charcoal in your diet and day-to-day routine can drastically improve the detoxification process as well.

Activated charcoal has the ability to block the absorption of harmful and hazardous compounds into the body while simultaneously absorbing and ridding the body of dangerous elements that were already present.

With 1 teaspoon of activated charcoal dissolved in 1 cup of water, you can detoxify the brain and body, resulting in more energy, improved cognitive functioning, increased immunity, and reduced incidences of illness and disease.

TOXICITY TODAY

With the current state of the world's environment being consistently polluted with the discharges of manufactured and synthetic products and the progressive degradation of the Earth's natural purifying capabilities, the air, water, and land around you is ever-changing in an unhealthy way. As a result of the barrage of toxins surrounding you every day, the need for detoxification can be a life-or-death situation. By removing impurities through treatments like those involving activated charcoal, you can safeguard your body and mind while preventing future health complications naturally!

15: TREATS SKIN IRRITATIONS

Among populations of all ages, skin irritations are a common occurrence. Whether the irritation is the result of an allergic reaction, environmental toxin, chemical, or organic compound, there are a wide variety of topical solutions available. These over-the-counter medications commonly contain synthetic additives and chemicals that can compound the existing irritation or extend the time period required to resolve the irritation, leading to serious side effects.

Nevertheless, redness, burning, sensitivity, pain, and swelling commonly coincide with the onset of a skin irritation, and topical solutions containing relieving elements can be helpful, but a one-two approach to resolving irritations that combines a topical and ingested solution can provide speedy relief and healing, as well as improved immunity.

Activated charcoal has the ability to absorb bacteria and microorganisms that can impede or agitate a skin irritation, and it can eliminate toxic components from both the skin's surface and from within the bloodstream. This dual approach to healing with activated charcoal not only prevents infection and irritation but can also provide pain relief and promote healing.

When the use of the following salve is combined with an ingested solution of 1 teaspoon of activated charcoal powder dissolved in a glass of water, the detoxifying substance can move through the body, be absorbed in the bloodstream, and activate within the digestive system in an effort to remove toxins and impurities that can contribute to the development of skin irritations or aggravate existing ones.

TO MAKE THE TOPICAL SALVE, COMBINE:

½–1 teaspoon activated charcoal powder
1 tablespoon water

Mix the ingredients well in a glass jar with a tight-fitting lid.

Apply to the irritated area and wrap with a bandage or mesh that can contain the salve until removed.

Redress every 2–4 hours.

16: TAKES THE STING OUT OF BUG BITES

Bug bites can range from mild (such as those from mosquitos) to possibly serious (such as stings from bees and wasps). A simple itchy bite can quickly lead to infection from scratching and breaking the skin, making it vulnerable to bacterial or viral infections. Bugs bites with venomous or poisonous secretions, as seen in bee and wasp stings, can create allergic reactions that lead to anaphylactic shock or decreased respiratory function. Some spider bites can even cause fatal reactions by compromising the cardiovascular, respiratory, and nervous systems.

With these considerations in mind, activated charcoal works as an effective and immediate treatment for bug bites and stings. It can be stored at home or carried easily for simple extraction of poisons and venom, as well as topical itch and pain relief applications. Because it contains absorbent and adsorbent abilities to extract and retain toxins from the body and bloodstream, activated charcoal can be used as an emergency bug bite treatment on people of any age without fear of side effects or complications.

TO MAKE A QUICK SALVE TO SOOTHE BUG BITES, USE:

½–1 teaspoon activated charcoal powder
1 tablespoon water

Combine the ingredients in a small bowl. Mix well.

Apply the salve topically to the site of the bug bite to alleviate pain, redness, irritation, burning, and swelling.

TO MAKE AN INGESTIBLE SOLUTION, USE:

1 teaspoon activated charcoal
1 cup water

Dissolve the activated charcoal in 1 cup of water and drink. This will help curb the flow of harsh poison or venom in the bloodstream, protecting the body from toxic overload and interference.

17: TREATS POISONING

Poisoning happens when a substance is ingested, inhaled, swallowed, injected, or absorbed through the skin, causing an adverse reaction that can result in severe harm or death. While the incidence of poisoning may seem rare, the prevalence of this extremely dangerous event is surprisingly high. In 2014, the American Association of Poison Control Centers (AAPCC) reported over 2.2 million human poison exposures, an average of one poisoning every 15 seconds. A shocking 48 percent of these poisonings were reported in children under the age of six, followed by 38 percent being reported in adults, and lastly with 7 percent being reported in teens. These incidences are classified in three categories:

Unintentional
- Therapeutic error
- Misuse
- Stings and bites
- Environmental
- Occupational
- Food

Intentional
- Suicide
- Misuse
- Abuse

Adverse Reactions
- Unexpected adverse reactions (such as allergies)

Poisoning occurs when toxic substances or harmful organic compounds bind and produce dangerous or deadly combinations that can interfere with, stress, halt, or negate the body's natural processes. This is best illustrated by anaphylactic reactions to poisoning, which cause the respiratory system to inflame and "shut down" following exposure to toxic chemical combinations, venom, stings, or environmental toxins.

Poisoning is a very serious situation and is commonly treated at local hospitals and emergency medical centers with activated charcoal. Able to absorb foreign chemicals and organic compounds effectively, activated charcoal is a safe method for relieving the body of poisonous elements and restoring natural balance and function to the body's organs and systems.

If you think you or someone else in your care has been poisoned, call 911 immediately.

18: TREATS BILE FLOW PROBLEMS IN PREGNANCY

According to the American Pregnancy Association, an estimated one out of every 1,000 pregnant women will experience a liver disease called cholestasis that only occurs during pregnancy. It is commonly seen in women with a family history of the disease, so a mother or sister who has been diagnosed will most likely have a female relative endure the same. It is also more widely reported among Swedish and Chilean women, as well as women who are carrying multiples or have previous liver damage. Most commonly, the onset of this disease occurs in the third trimester and usually goes away within the first few days following delivery.

Cholestasis renders the gallbladder, which stores the bile produced by the liver for the digestion of fats, unable to efficiently release its stores of bile into the small intestine. Whether there is inflammation of the ducts or a complete blockage, bile begins to buildup in the gallbladder and can spill into the bloodstream. The most frequently reported symptom is a severe itchiness that can be described as being "under or in the skin." Other symptoms include:

- Fatigue
- Weight loss
- Brown urine
- Greasy stools
- Loss of appetite
- Night sweats
- Fever
- Yellowing of the skin

The concern with this disease is that the unborn baby can be at serious risk for fetal distress, preterm delivery, or even stillbirth. A doctor can diagnose cholestasis quickly through a previous medical history analysis, physical exam, and blood test. Once diagnosed, activated charcoal can be used simply and safely to absorb and remove the harsh metals, built-up minerals, inflammatory compounds, and coagulated organic material that can all contribute to the blocking of the gallbladder's bile ducts. With absolutely no risk to the baby, a pregnant woman with cholestasis can effectively reduce the incidence of bile flow issues with a simple teaspoon of activated charcoal mixed with water and consumed daily until symptoms subside and liver and gallbladder functions return to normal.

19: PREVENTS DRUG OVERDOSES

Defined as an ingestion or application of a drug or substance in a quantity greater than recommended or regularly practiced, drug overdoses are described by the Centers for Disease Control and Prevention as a condition that can lead to a toxic state or death. Because the symptoms of drug overdose vary depending on the drug or substance that was used in excess, it can be difficult to determine the best measures to take in order to save an overdose victim's life. Medical professionals communicate with an overdose victim in hopes of being able to determine the cause as quickly as possible, or they may have to determine the cause without the patient's assistance in situations where the patient is incapacitated, unresponsive, or unconscious.

The most common treatment for overdoses since the 1960s has been activated charcoal. Binding with foreign agents, chemicals, and compounds in the bloodstream and digestive system, activated charcoal has been viewed as the safest course of action when treating overdoses. Not only has activated charcoal been deemed most effective in saving an overdose patient's life, but the success rate when it is administered within an hour of an overdose has been impressive, even by medical standards. While other forms of medications can be used, these synthetic prescriptions and invasive treatments can cause serious side effects or severe bodily harm to the patient. In lieu of up-and-coming pharmaceutical and invasive "purging" treatments, most medical professionals utilize the absorptive and adsorptive abilities of activated charcoal more readily, hoping to save the lives of the thousands of overdose victims that succumb to excessive drug exposure every year.

20: PREVENTS POISONING IN CHILDREN

The Centers for Disease Control and Prevention and the American Association of Poison Control Centers have determined that an estimated 300 children are treated for some form of poisoning daily, with an average of two deaths each day. With household cleaners, pesticides, chemical formulations, and cosmetics being commonplace in the average American household, the consistent rise in annual childhood poisonings is not surprising. The colorful packaging and eye-catching marketing ploys that are used to attract parents to certain products can have the same appeal to small children who are unaware of the harmful or even deadly ingredient formulations inside. A number of laundry detergent manufacturers came under fire in 2012 for their product packaging of single-use detergent packets. The colorful, squishy, bite-sized packets were packaged in clear candy-bowl shaped containers, and the number of children who were mistakenly ingesting laundry detergent quickly skyrocketed, with 4,868 children being poisoned in the first half of 2013 alone.

While the statistics related to childhood poisoning are alarming, there are steps that can be taken to minimize the chances of an incident in your home:

1. Keep the number for poison control readily available: (800) 222-1222
2. Lock up all chemicals and hazardous organic materials
3. Store any unlocked chemicals out of children's reach
4. Dispose of unnecessary or unused chemicals
5. Read labels carefully to determine the safety risks of household products

In cases of childhood poisoning, activated charcoal is almost always utilized because it is safe and has a promising success rate. Activated charcoal can absorb most poisonous chemicals or harmful organic compounds and restore a natural balance to the digestive system and bloodstream, thereby preventing any adverse physical and mental ramifications of poisoning.

SEEK MEDICAL HELP

If you suspect someone, especially a child, has ingested some poisonous material you need to get professional medical advice. Always seek emergency medical treatment immediately for any cases of poisoning or suspected poisoning.

21: ALLEVIATES PSORIASIS

Approximately 7.5 million people in the US have psoriasis. Psoriasis is an incurable condition that is persistent, unpredictable, and irritating to the extent that it can interfere with daily life. The disease causes skin cells to produce at a rapid rate (more than ten times the normal production speed), resulting in raised, red, scaly, itchy, dry patches that can appear on any part of the skin's surface. While topical creams and ointments, oral medications, and light therapies can be used to minimize the condition, few of these treatments provide long-lasting relief. Furthermore, the physical conditions that can result from the onset of psoriasis flare-ups include joint pain, tendonitis, stress, depression, anxiety, and fatigue. With all of these physical and psychological ramifications of psoriasis, it's no wonder that the medical and holistic communities have strived to determine an effective treatment.

Studies have been performed to determine if activated charcoal can be utilized in the successful treatment of psoriasis, and each has shown promise. The underlying cause of psoriasis development has been traced back to bacterial toxins that poison the liver and blood, aggravating the immune system and contributing to inflammation. Activated charcoal is able to travel through the bloodstream and digestive system, removing these toxins and impurities to provide the liver with relief.

The most commonly studied treatment regimen is not only topical (please see the salve recipe in entry 33) but also includes an oral application of 2½ teaspoons of activated charcoal dissolved in water and consumed in three smaller, separate dosages. By topically providing relief and internally ridding the body of the toxins responsible for the disease, activated charcoal can be an effective, safe, all-natural treatment for any psoriasis sufferer.

22: TREATS SENSITIVITY IN TEETH

By restricting the diet to only hot or cold foods, interfering with normal oral hygiene, or even impairing basic functions like talking and eating, tooth sensitivity is a serious issue that millions of people struggle with every day. Excessive brushing, chronic indigestion, eating disorders, and countless other health conditions and associated medications can all contribute to the deterioration of the protective enamel and dentin that keep the sensitive root of each tooth safe.

While tooth decay and cavities can contribute to sensitive teeth, the more common culprits are mineral deficiencies and the chronic deterioration of enamel. There are countless oral health products that promise to deliver relief from tooth sensitivity, but these products are often packed with harsh chemicals and synthetic additives. Not only are these products unpredictable, but their focus on the exterior of the teeth neglects the mineral metabolism that the body requires to retain essential dentin and enamel.

By utilizing activated charcoal in oral and ingested applications, you can return your mouth to a healthy balance, naturally restoring the essential minerals in the bloodstream and body. Activated charcoal will also support your oral health maintenance systems that produce saliva, eliminate bad bacteria, and retain minerals within the teeth.

Using an activated charcoal toothpaste and mouthwash in conjunction with 1 teaspoon of activated charcoal in meals, smoothies, or solutions each day will help alleviate tooth sensitivity easily and naturally.

TO MAKE A TOOTHPASTE, USE:

½ teaspoon activated charcoal powder
½ teaspoon water

Combine both ingredients to form a paste. Use to brush teeth as normal.

TO MAKE MOUTHWASH, USE:

½ teaspoon activated charcoal powder
1 tablespoon water

Combine both ingredients and swish around mouth to rinse. Spit out mixture.

23: TRAPS IMPURITIES IN WATER

Water contamination is a worldwide problem that affects lakes, rivers, oceans, aquifers, and groundwater, contributing to a global health crisis that is estimated to adversely affect millions around the world. Waterborne diseases are actually responsible for claiming the lives of 14,000 people every day. While it may seem logical that this issue would be exclusive to underdeveloped countries and communities, many water sources in developed and affluent countries struggle with water pollution as well.

When chemicals, organic compounds, and harmful pathogens flood waterways and water resources, some treatment applications utilize harsh chemicals like chlorine to "cleanse" the water and make it acceptable for consumption. This compounding of health-compromising chemicals, additives, and organic materials not only deteriorates the natural processes throughout the body but can also seriously compromise the health of organs and systems on which the body relies.

Due to its absorbent and adsorbent qualities, activated charcoal is the most commonly used product in water filtration processes. Because it has the capability to attract countless chemicals and organic compounds, charcoal can filter disease-causing elements from water naturally. Effective, inexpensive, and readily available, activated charcoal is being increasingly implemented in filtration systems in homes and communities across the globe.

To conduct a simple filtration of questionable water, use 1 tablespoon of activated charcoal per 5 gallons of water, or you can insert a "brick" of activated charcoal weighing 25 grams into a water delivery system to naturally reduce the incidence of health issues on a larger scale.

24: PREVENTS THE GROWTH OF MOLD

Over the past few decades, research and scientific studies have determined the dangers of mold. A common fungus that can grow indoors and out, mold is thought to have between 10,000 and 300,000 species. Infiltrating homes, outdoor areas, plants and gardens, and even workplaces, concern about mold's impact on health has grown steadily in recent years.

Reactions to mold are usually similar to common allergic reactions… but with far more harmful health consequences. Nasal stuffiness, eye irritation, wheezing, and skin irritations are just the mild symptoms of mold exposure. More severe reactions include the development of asthmatic symptoms such as shortness of breath, fever, lung infections, headaches, and fatigue. In children, consistent mold exposure can contribute to the development of serious upper respiratory infections and chronic illness. With these serious health threats, the removal of mold is obviously a high priority for most individuals.

As opposed to the common mold-killing solution of 1 cup of water and 1 cup of bleach, activated charcoal can serve as an effective, all-natural treatment for ridding any space of fungal growth. Make a paste as follows and apply the organic, absorptive mixture to any area. After it is rinsed away thoroughly, the activated charcoal can fight existing mold while also providing preventative protection against future mold growth safely and naturally.

TO MAKE A MOLD-FIGHTING PASTE, USE:

½ cup activated charcoal powder
1 cup water

Combine both ingredients and mix well to form a paste.

Apply to the area infected with mold and allow it to set for 10–20 minutes.

Rinse area thoroughly.

25: REDUCES JOINT PAIN

Chronic joint pain is caused by inflammation that inhibits the fluid movement of the joints in any part of the body, resulting in limited mobility, less physical exercise, depression and anxiety, and often unemployment. While there are a growing number of medications intended to treat inflammation of the joints and minimize joint pain, these medications can be packed with synthetic chemicals and additives that pose serious risks to a patient's health.

Because this condition has become more prevalent among all age groups (even children), finding the underlying cause has been a major focus of scientific studies in recent years. With inflammation being identified as the preexisting condition that most contributes to swelling, immobility, and joint pain, treatments that improve nutrition, increase physical activity, and reduce injury, illness, and disease are needed to help limit inflammatory responses in the body.

Medications are the most common treatment for arthritis and joint pain, but activated charcoal has been found in studies to have a similar (if not more effective) success rate in the treatment of these conditions. Activated charcoal can purge the bloodstream of impurities, cleanse the joints, muscles, and tendons of toxic substances, and restore the natural mineral balance that's essential for overall health. A simple ingestion of 1 teaspoon of activated charcoal dissolved in 1 cup of water daily, in conjunction with a topical salve (see recipe in entry 33) that can be applied directly to painful joints, provides an all-natural strategy for restoring joint mobility and improving overall health.

26: REDUCES LIVER DAMAGE

The liver plays a major role in a number of the body's systems and processes. The liver's main job is to filter the blood from the digestive tract before passing it to the rest of the body. It also detoxifies chemicals, metabolizes drugs, and makes proteins that are important for blood clotting and other functions. When liver failure occurs, the results can be catastrophic. Liver failure can be acute, occurring rapidly in as little as forty-eight hours, or it can progress gradually over the course of years. Illness and disease are the most common contributors to liver damage, but there are a number of other factors that can affect the liver's cells, including:

- Hepatitis B
- Hepatitis C
- Long-term alcohol abuse
- Excessive iron absorption (hemochromatosis)
- Malnutrition

With any or all of these conditions contributing to diminished liver function, many patients experience a common set of symptoms that indicate the liver is failing to perform optimally. Nausea, loss of appetite, fatigue, diarrhea, jaundice, difficulty clotting or profuse bleeding, abnormal bloating of the abdomen, and even disorientation and confusion can all result from faulty liver function.

Most physicians will recommend a combination of lifestyle changes and medication, but the medications commonly prescribed can have serious side effects that compromise the body's systems, aggravate inflammation, or even produce new symptoms that adversely affect the body and mind.

With an all-natural approach to ridding the liver of toxins and impurities, activated charcoal can be utilized as an effective treatment method for liver cells damaged by illness, disease, or unhealthy lifestyle habits. One teaspoon of activated charcoal combined with food or consumed in a solution of 1 cup of water can restore liver cell health naturally.

27: PROMOTES COGNITIVE FUNCTIONING

Cognitive functioning refers to all of the mental processes that occur within the nervous system and brain, such as thought processing, memory, and recognition. These everyday brain activities that allow you to recognize your surroundings, pay attention, remember people, places, and things, and recount your daily to-dos can easily be taken for granted...until they're compromised by illness, disease, malnutrition, old age, injury, and so on. Even commonly prescribed medications can have a lasting effect on brain functioning that adversely affects cognitive processes.

While brain games, improved nutrition, regular exercise, and abstinence from drugs and alcohol can all help in the maintenance of cognitive functioning, the optimization of cognitive processes relies on the removal of toxic elements, chemicals, and organic compounds that can interfere with the brain's ability to successfully communicate with other areas of the body. When the blood, body, and brain are cleansed of these inhibiting elements, ideal cognitive functioning can be restored naturally.

Free of the unhealthy side effects that can result from repeated use of medications, 1 teaspoon of activated charcoal can be consumed in daily meals and in a simple solution mixed with 1 cup of water to help safeguard the brain's health and promote healthy cognitive functioning for years to come.

THE IMPORTANCE OF INFORMATION RETAINMENT

When the brain functions normally, information is able to be introduced and retained short-term or long-term. With the constant degradation of the brain's capabilities that results from age, toxicity, or illness, the brain and mind can become compromised over time. Adding activated charcoal to your daily regimen in addition to brain exercises that challenge the brain's processes and procedures, you can help your brain retain information, improve thought processing, and safeguard cognitive capabilities throughout life.

28: SUPPORTS HEALTHY ADRENAL GLAND FUNCTIONING

Located at the top of the kidneys, the walnut-sized adrenal glands are unassuming in appearance and weigh less than a grape. These small organs may seem insignificant in size, but they play a major role in a number of the body's functions and processes. Responsible for essential hormone production and processing, the adrenal glands affect everything from metabolism to processing and absorbing essential micro- and macronutrients to sleep patterns and stress levels.

Chronic conditions, illnesses, and diseases can wreak havoc on the adrenal glands, causing an over- or underproduction of the hormones on which the entire body and brain heavily rely. The most common conditions that interfere with adrenal functioning are chronic stress, excessive alcohol consumption, drug use (medicinal and illicit), poor diet and lifestyle habits, obesity, and diabetes.

Poor adrenal gland functioning can cause blood sugar spikes and dips, high blood pressure, poor metabolic functioning, weight gain and weight loss, increased or depleted energy levels, interrupted sleep or chronic fatigue, and an over- or underproduction of essential sex hormones.

A number of studies and research programs that have explored the effectiveness of alternative, holistic approaches to medicinal therapies for adrenal gland malfunctioning have focused on activated charcoal. When consumed orally, a single serving of 1–3 teaspoons daily dissolved in 1 cup of water, activated charcoal showed a promising effect on adrenal gland functions. If you feel your adrenal gland functioning may be less than ideal and is contributing to symptoms that interfere with your daily life, try incorporating activated charcoal in your daily diet for quick, all-natural restoration of health.

29: TREATS ALCOHOL POISONING

According to the Centers for Disease Control and Prevention, alcohol poisoning causes six deaths daily in America. While alcohol consumption is a socially acceptable practice, the regularly displayed characteristics and behaviors associated with alcohol poisoning are almost always gently referred to as "drunkenness." Slurred speech, lack of coordination, and mood and behavioral changes are just a few symptoms associated with the onset of alcohol poisoning. The more serious symptoms that appear as the severity of alcohol poisoning progresses are:

1. Aggression
2. Amnesia
3. Blackout
4. Clammy skin
5. Confusion
6. Dehydration
7. Depression
8. Euphoria
9. Flushing
10. Nausea
11. Seizures
12. Stupor
13. Unconsciousness
14. Uncontrollable rapid eye movements
15. Unresponsiveness
16. Vomiting

When any of these symptoms occur following the consumption of four or more drinks for women or five or more drinks for men, the probability of alcohol poisoning is high. Age, gender, diet, previous history of alcohol consumption or abuse, genetics, and race are just a few factors that can affect an individual's ability to process alcohol efficiently. Compounding these factors are medication consumption (prescribed or otherwise), gastrointestinal difficulties, kidney or liver illness or disease, and stress, anxiety, and depression levels. With all these variables playing a role in an individual's ability to process alcohol effectively, it's easy to see why individual experiences with alcohol vary so much from person to person and sometimes result in alcohol poisoning.

While emergency medical professionals should be called immediately if alcohol poisoning is suspected, the administration of activated charcoal upon diagnosis is essential for absorbing toxic elements within the digestive system and bloodstream and quickly returning the body and brain to a stable condition. With the assistance of medical professionals', emergency personnel's, or poison control professionals' instructions, life-saving action implementing activated charcoal can be administered while awaiting emergency assistance if necessary. If instructed to proceed with interventions using activated charcoal, the medical professionals who are providing instructions will provide the necessary information referring to the dosage amount and administration procedures depending on the victim's weight, consumption of toxic substances, and so on.

Because one of the benefits of activated charcoal focuses on the detoxification and purification of the cells, organs, and systems, the use of activated charcoal powder can help rid the system of alcohol, build-up of bile, and harmful toxic reactions that can occur throughout the body as a result of overdose of any synthetic or natural element that causes discomfort or contributes to chronic conditions or illnesses.

30: CLEANSES BLOOD

Millions of people worldwide experience health complications related to blood disorders every year. Chronic conditions, illness, disease, wounds, surgeries, and common immune system complications can all leave the body at risk for developing a blood infection or condition that can lead to severe blood toxicity. Sepsis and septicemia are the two most common conditions that affect the bloodstream and can compromise the health, or life, of a patient. Disguised by flu-like symptoms, blood toxemia conditions can be hard to diagnose without a medical professional's analysis. Symptoms such as fever, rapid or slowed breathing, rapid or slowed heartbeat, paleness, confusion, and little or no urine production can all be indications that a blood disorder is to blame.

While a number of medical treatments can be administered in an attempt to return the normal balance within the bloodstream, these medications and treatments can have debilitating side effects that complicate existing health conditions or cause the development of new ones. In the presence of normally harmless bacteria and viruses, patients with a compromised immune system can easily have their blood cells overtaken with infection, leading to diminished blood health. Pathogens and illness-causing bacteria and viruses can move out of the bloodstream and also infect organs, tissues, and cells.

Activated charcoal has a number of absorbent qualities that allow it to travel through the bloodstream, body, and brain, absorbing toxins, chemicals, and compounds that can put blood health at risk. Due to its ability to combat the infiltration of bacterial, viral, and fungal infections, activated charcoal can be used as a preventative and curative measure safely and naturally.

31: SOOTHES SORE THROATS

Among all ages, genders, and backgrounds, a sore throat is one of the most commonly reported condition. While the usual causes of a sore throat are related to bacterial and viral infections, other causes, including smoking, overuse of the voice (yelling or straining vocal chords for extended periods of time), allergies, a compromised immune system, consuming excessively hot foods, and even sleeping with the mouth open. Young children and the elderly are the most common groups to report this condition, but a sore throat can strike any patient of any age.

While a number of pain relievers and medications are available to treat the inflammation and infections associated with the onset of sore throats, a number of these medications either prove to be ineffective, complicate other preexisting conditions, or exacerbate the sore throat by increasing inflammatory responses or causing serious side effects.

The oral ingestion of a simple teaspoon of activated charcoal dissolved in 1 cup of warm water can be used in combination with other treatment methods, including gargling with the solution, brushing the teeth and mouth with the solution, or simply consuming the solution to fend off the bacteria, virus, chemical imbalance, or inflammatory compounds that are contributing to the development of sore throat symptoms.

TO MAKE A THROAT-SOOTHING ACTIVATED CHARCOAL TEA, FOLLOW THESE STEPS:

1 cup hot water
1 green tea bag
1 teaspoon freshly squeezed lemon juice
½–1 teaspoon activated charcoal powder

In a mug, combine water, tea bag, and lemon juice. Stir and allow to cool slightly for 5 minutes.

Remove tea bag and stir activated charcoal into water until well blended.

Sip the tea, stirring as needed to prevent activated charcoal from settling at the bottom of the mug.

32: ALLEVIATES ALLERGIES

Every year in the United States, an estimated 50 million Americans suffer from some type of allergy. While allergic reactions to foods, bites and stings, dust, and pollen are the most commonly reported, there are a number of environmental, situational, and physical conditions that contribute to an allergic reaction in the body. Whether the reaction is red and itchy eyes, a runny nose, congestion, difficulty breathing, coughing, or even indigestion, allergic reactions can cause serious physical reactions that can interfere with daily life.

The most common allergy symptoms can create cognitive interference, such as difficulty focusing, mental fatigue, energy depletion, physical exhaustion, and even flu-like symptoms that can encompass chest pain, nausea, vomiting, muscle soreness, and body aches. These inflammatory responses that attack the brain, respiratory system, and musculoskeletal system can all be attributed to allergens infiltrating the bloodstream and acting as pathogens disrupting the body's normal systematic functions and processes.

Activated charcoal can be used as a purging agent, traveling safely through the bloodstream, digestive system, and body to attract and trap the impurities, toxins, and volatile organic compounds that contribute to allergic reactions. When these allergens are removed from the body's systems, the natural stability of metabolic, hormonal, and cardiovascular system functions is restored, helping resolve respiratory, cognitive, and digestive issues.

A simple teaspoon of activated charcoal consumed in a solution of 1 cup of water can alleviate allergy symptoms within thirty to sixty minutes and help block allergens for twenty-four hours. Because the product is all-natural, activated charcoal has no harmful side effects, additives, or preservatives that can complicate existing conditions.

33: REDUCES MUSCLE SORENESS

Muscle soreness can result from a number of scenarios, including exertion, overuse, stretching or tearing of muscle tissues, injury, illness, disease, drug use, or malnutrition. Whether the cause is a buildup of lactic acid (a natural by-product produced from exercising a muscle or muscle group) or fibromyalgia (a disease that affects muscles and nerve cells, causing muscular pain), muscle soreness can cause serious discomfort.

Because the condition can interfere with the ability to move freely, muscle soreness in daily life can be very severe, especially for the elderly population. Additionally, chronic conditions that contribute to immobility, such as joint stiffness, arthritis, and injury, can grow worse with inactivity. Luckily, activated charcoal can provide a treatment regimen that is simple, safe, and effective.

Along with simple stretching exercises that target sore muscles, you should try a two-step activated charcoal treatment. First, create a topical salve using the first of the following recipes and apply it to the sore area. The topical application helps withdraw toxins and impurities from the skin and bloodstream. Next, consume an ingested form of activated charcoal according to the second recipe. This solution can travel through the digestive system and bloodstream, effectively removing toxins and impurities that can contribute to muscle soreness. This one-two punch can help support muscle health while minimizing soreness naturally!

TO MAKE THE TOPICAL SALVE, USE:

1 tablespoon activated charcoal powder
1 tablespoon water

Combine the ingredients into a paste and apply to the sore muscle area. Wrap in gauze and then plastic wrap and leave on 4–6 hours.

TO MAKE THE INGESTED CHARCOAL, USE:

1 cup of water
1 teaspoon activated charcoal powder

Mix the ingredients well and drink immediately.

34: NATURALLY RELIEVES PAIN

Pain relievers are a common over-the-counter medication that can help alleviate a patient's suffering. While readily available and commonly prescribed, these medications can fail to provide adequate relief, cause serious side effects, and even contribute to severe illness and disease.

Acetaminophen is one of the most commonly prescribed pain relievers, but it's the biggest contributor to the development of liver disease...even more so than alcohol abuse! With the extensive filtration that's required of the body's organs to process, distribute, and flush these medications throughout the body, pain relief seems to come at a cost most aren't willing to pay. The sacrifice of overall long-term health for short-term relief doesn't equate. Luckily, natural healing communities and medical professionals have found activated charcoal is an effective alternative to pain relievers.

Purging the body of inflammatory compounds that can contribute to pain and discomfort in bones, muscles, tissues, and joints, activated charcoal attracts, absorbs, and transports pain-causing elements out of the body. Providing the same cleansing benefits to the bloodstream, brain, and digestive system, the activated charcoal can remove chemicals, compounds, and organic elements that interfere with the body's natural processes, thereby improving immunity, support system functioning, and healthy hormone production, all of which help minimize infection, inflammation, and illness that can contribute to pain. With a simple solution of 1 teaspoon of activated charcoal combined with a glass of water, any patient in need of pain relief can put aside their potentially harmful, chemical-laden drugs and medicines and rely on this risk-free, all-natural treatment instead.

35: IMPROVES BONE HEALTH

Every year, countless patients suffer from conditions related to deteriorated bone health. In fact every year approximately 1.5 million individuals suffer a fracture due to bone disease.

The bones are essential to storing important vitamins and minerals, particularly calcium and phosphorous, that contribute proper system functioning throughout the body. The skeletal structures also support and protect the body's organs. When the bones are compromised with illness, disease, and malnutrition, the body's systems react accordingly, leading to a continuous cycle of nutrient depletion and imbalance. By taking certain precautionary measures, making changes in lifestyle habits, and improving dietary intake, the risk of developing conditions that can contribute to the deterioration of bone health can be minimized naturally.

Activated charcoal can help reduce the risk of bone health issues effectively, naturally, and easily. It has porous characteristics that give it the ability to attract and trap impurities and pathogens that can contribute to the deterioration of bone health. When certain toxins, organic compounds, and disturbed levels of hormones, enzymes, and nutrients become aggravated or imbalanced, the bones can suffer major distress. Activated charcoal protects the mineral composition of bones, helping the skeletal framework remain intact.

Activated charcoal also assists in bone health preservation by removing harmful elements that can wreak havoc on bone health. A single serving (or 1 teaspoon) of activated charcoal in a glass of water can provide natural relief that supports the bones, the body, and the brain.

36: DEPLETES DEPRESSIVE CONDITIONS

An estimated 15 million Americans suffer from major depressive disorder according to the Anxiety and Depression Association of America. Depression is a serious medical condition that can severely affect and alter the quality of life of its sufferers and should be addressed as soon as possible to prevent negative or even potentially deadly outcomes.

With an appropriate diagnosis, depression sufferers can find relief and resolve the underlying issues that may have contributed to the development of their disorder. Unfortunately, they can also fall victim to countless side effects that stem from prescription antidepressant medications. The risk of suicidal thoughts and actions that accompanies many prescribed medications for depression has triggered an outcry for more effective therapies and methods of treatment.

Activated charcoal has the ability to purge harmful toxins from the bloodstream, brain, and body that can convolute the systems and processes responsible for essential hormone production and balance. While supporting the brain's neurotransmitters and boosting the systems that can alleviate stress, support cognitive functioning, and aid in healthy metabolic functioning of essential nutrients, activated charcoal can act as an effective treatment method for depression without the risk of side effects. A serving of 1 teaspoon of activated charcoal dissolved in 1 cup of water can be consumed one to three times daily until the brain and body are restored to their natural state. This dosage will also help promote and maintain optimal systematic functioning of all glands, organs, and systems related to the processes responsible for depressive disorders.

TRY LIFESTYLE CHANGES FOR DEPRESSION

There are countless medications available for depressive disorders, but they often lead to heavily medicated patients who achieve little or no improvements in their symptoms. By opting for healthier lifestyle choices that focus on diet, sleep, exercise, and refraining from depression-inducing alcohol and drugs, the average person can combat their depression symptoms naturally.

37: REDUCES INCIDENCES OF GINGIVITIS

Gingivitis has become an increasingly concerning problem for a majority of Americans. There are many campaigns designed to emphasize the need for oral healthcare, regular dental visits, and awareness about the serious health issues that can result from neglectful oral care. Unfortunately, there is also a barrage of commercial marketing messages playing off that healthcare advice, claiming disinfecting mouthwashes, expensive toothbrushes, and excessive toothcare accessories are the answer to oral care. While the expensive varieties of toothpastes, mouth rinses, and preventative products may seem enticing to the well-intentioned consumer, many of these products leave chemicals, synthetic materials, and harsh additives in the mouth that can aggravate existing conditions or even contribute to the development of new ones.

By using a charcoal paste that combines a ½ teaspoon of activated charcoal with a ½ teaspoon of water, anyone can brush their teeth clean of viruses, bacteria, and harmful organic compounds that can deteriorate oral health. In addition, a solution of 1 teaspoon of activated charcoal combined with 1 cup of water can be consumed daily to combat the bacterial, viral, and volatile organic compounds that can breed inside the body and contribute to undesirable oral health conditions.

By introducing activated charcoal to the teeth, gums, and tongue, as well as throughout the digestive system, you can help boost the curative and preventative properties that not only safeguard oral health but also banish the unhealthy toxicity that can contribute to the development of gingivitis.

Every year, 16 million visits to medical professionals are due to sinus issues, 1 billion dollars are spent to treat the conditions, and over 150 million dollars are spent on prescriptions and medications related to the treatment. The sinuses are air-filled cavities that lie within the upper cheeks, behind the forehead, on either side of the nose, and directly in front of the brain. When there are disruptions in the sinus cavities from allergies, asthma, blockages, or illness and disease, the symptoms that result can be as mild as an over-production of mucus and stuffiness to severe reactions that include headaches, tooth pain, facial pain, and bad breath. When patients suffer from sinus conditions regularly, or even multiple times in the same year, an ear, nose, and throat specialist can determine if continuing prescription treatment is healthier than treating the condition with surgical intervention.

In lieu of repetitive antibiotic or surgical treatments that can wreak havoc on the overall health and well-being of a sinus-infection sufferer, activated charcoal provides the body with antibacterial, antimicrobial, antifungal, and anti-inflammatory benefits that can directly combat the underlying causes of sinus issues. Purging the bloodstream, respiratory system, and sinuses of impurities, allergens, and inflammatory compounds, 1 teaspoon of ingested activated charcoal (dissolved in 1 cup of water or food) provides all-natural relief and preventative benefits too.

SINUS ISSUES THAT INDICATE INFECTION

Because the sinuses impact the majority of the facial area, an astounding number of symptoms can result from an infection in the sinus cavities. Pain, aches, and throbbing, such as headaches and toothaches, can all be the result of an infection in the sinuses. A fever or other associated symptoms can be a sign to start a sinus-healing treatment like activated charcoal…not only to improve the health of the sinuses but also the health of the entire body.

39: INCREASES ENERGY LEVELS

One of the most widely searched terms on the Internet relating to health doesn't involve specific conditions or symptoms; it involves energy levels and (more specifically) how to increase energy. With all the caffeine, energy drinks, and stimulant products that are consumed every day by millions of Americans, the need for increased energy is more apparent than ever. Marketers of these products try to convince consumers that they can have the energy they need without taking the time to address the underlying cause of the reduced energy levels they are experiencing. Whether the contributing factor is a poor diet, illness or disease, lack of sleep, anxiety or depression, or any of a multitude of interrupted physical processes that naturally contribute to the production of energy in the body and mind, lack of energy cannot be cured with a single-serving pill, potion, or application that merely masks the underlying issue temporarily.

With the regular consumption of activated charcoal, the body can purge itself of toxins and impurities that contribute to the degradation of organs and systems that are responsible for energy production. By consuming 1 teaspoon of activated charcoal dissolved in 1 cup of water daily, anyone experiencing reduced energy levels can enjoy a multitude of rejuvenating health benefits that not only maintain and improve energy but also help improve and safeguard the overall health of the entire body and mind.

THE DANGER OF ENERGY DRINKS

Energy drinks are growing more prominent and popular with each passing year. These energy-spiking drinks can be packed with caffeine, harmful herbs, or synthetic additives that can complicate the body's natural processes or even cause a catastrophic spike and drop in energy levels. By opting for natural solutions, such as committing to a clean diet, consuming naturally energizing drinks like teas, and exercising more, anyone can utilize healthy habits and improve energy naturally without taking any risks.

40: PROMOTES NERVE FUNCTIONING

When the body is healthy and the nervous system is able to function as intended, it can be easy to take proper nerve functioning for granted. Most of us fail to realize how important a healthy nervous system truly is. Every thought we think, word we speak, or action we take is the result of messages that are clearly and concisely relayed from one nerve network to another. When these networks become convoluted or damaged, cognitive processing, mood, behavior, speech, and motor control can all be adversely affected, having a major impact on quality of life.

The most commonly diagnosed nervous system impairments, aside from those resulting from injury, are due to a chemical imbalance that results from toxicity. When volatile organic compounds, chemicals, and other damaging illnesses or diseases barrage the body and brain, the degradation of nervous cells and networks can be extreme enough to interrupt the networks' communication with one another. Therapies and medications can be prescribed in an effort to restore healthy nerve function, but their potential for ineffectiveness and possible side effects can outweigh the possible benefits.

The daily consumption of 1 teaspoon of activated charcoal dissolved in 1 cup of water can help prevent nerve damage and promote healthy nervous system functioning safely and naturally. With the ability to move through the body, brain, and bloodstream, absorbing and removing harmful toxins that can attack the nerves, activated charcoal is able to cleanse impurities, restore an optimal balance of nutrients and hormones that support nerve health, and maintain an optimal level of nerve system network communication. Simple and easy, a daily dose of activated charcoal can safeguard and support the body and mind from nervous system failure, ensuring an active life for years to come!

41: IMPROVES MEMORY

The memory plays such an important role in life that its maintenance is imperative. Helping to retain past experiences, thoughts, and feelings, and guiding us through everyday activities that make enjoyable life possible, the memory is an essential part of the brain. However, illness, disease, and chronic conditions can quickly result in physical and mental complications that degrade memories and compromise the brain's ability to retain information. As a result, the awareness of preventative and proactive measures to safeguard memory is increasing in medical and natural health communities around the world.

With daily exercise, mental "workouts" and brain games, adequate sleep, stress reduction, proper nutrition, and positive improvements in lifestyle habits that affect health, the cognitive functions that help maintain memory and reduce the risk of memory loss can be safeguarded naturally. The consumption of activated charcoal can make maintaining memory easy.

Activated charcoal provides the body with protection against pathogens, organic compounds, chemicals, and toxins that can negatively affect energy levels, immunity, metabolic processes, and cognitive functioning. It acts as both a preventative measure and an element of support for the functions and processes keeping the body and mind free of damaging toxicity that threatens the well-being of our memory.

42: MINIMIZES MORNING SICKNESS

Most pregnant women experience some form of morning sickness during their ten-month-long adventure of pregnancy. Regardless of the mother's age, race, weight, or the gender of the baby, morning sickness symptoms like nausea, dizziness, lightheadedness, food aversions, heartburn, indigestion, and vomiting can occur in any pregnancy.

With the hormonal fluctuations that are inevitable in the development of a healthy baby, morning sickness can happen at any point (day or night). While old wives' tales claim that morning sickness is caused by an unborn baby's physical attributes (like hair length or eye color) or personality, the true underlying causes can be credited to hormonal imbalances and upsets in the digestive system.

While a number of medications can be prescribed in an effort to minimize the severity or prevalence of morning sickness, many contain chemical formulations that can trigger serious side effects and produce complications to the mom or unborn baby. Even all-natural treatments can create dangerous situations, because certain vitamins, drinks, and herbal therapies are not approved as safe for consumption during pregnancy.

Activated charcoal has been approved by almost every obstetrical organization and has even been deemed safe by the Food and Drug Administration. With the consumption of 1 teaspoon of activated charcoal dissolved in 1 cup of water, pregnant women can find natural relief from heartburn, indigestion, stomach upsets, nausea, and vomiting without fear of harsh side effects or dangers posed to the baby.

43: NATURALLY IMPROVES APPETITE

Weight loss can sometimes be seen as a positive if weight is an issue aesthetically or medically, but when an individual's weight is low to begin with, the loss of appetite and aversion to foods can seriously compromise the body's cells, organs, and systems that rely on quality nutrients for proper functioning. Whether appetite loss is the result of illness, disease, stress, anxiety, depression, or even common medications, the complications that can occur throughout the body and brain as a result of insufficient nutrition can be disastrous.

An individual who suffers from loss of appetite is in danger of compromised functioning of essential systems and possibly even failure of important organs. Through a number of therapeutic interventions and medical testing, the underlying cause of appetite loss can be determined, but activated charcoal can also help restore appetite and balance to the body and brain while other contributing factors are addressed.

Helping to purge the body and brain of inorganic and organic compounds, toxins, and harsh elements that contribute to illnesses affecting the appetite, activated charcoal can aid in the recovery from common conditions that make individuals nauseated or sick to their stomach. Restoring balance to the systems that contribute to digestion, cognitive processing, neural communication, blood health, and immunity, a single teaspoon of activated charcoal dissolved in 1 cup of water daily can naturally stimulate the body's processes and encourage the return of a healthy appetite.

44: IMPROVES FUNCTIONING OF THE CARDIOVASCULAR SYSTEM

The cardiovascular system is one of the most important systems of the body, consisting of the heart, blood vessels, and blood. When the cardiovascular system's functioning is compromised, the results can be catastrophic or even deadly. Age, genetics, diet, lifestyle habits, exposure to harmful elements, weight, and blood sugar levels are all potential risk factors for diminished cardiovascular function over time without proper attention and treatment. Modern medicinal approaches can diagnose and specify the appropriate treatment methods for a specific cardiovascular condition. For instance, an individual with a situation relating to the arteries, blood health, blood flow, or overall performance of the heart can receive necessary medical advice, treatment, and counseling on future preventative measures they can take to reduce their risk of a stroke, heart attack, or death.

Every day, 2,000 gallons of blood travel throughout 60,000 miles of vessels that comprise the cardiovascular system. When the heart, arteries, or vessels become clogged, obstructed, or damaged, the minimized flow of essential oxygenated blood to the organs snowballs into a repetitive cycle that puts those organs' functions at risk. With the daily consumption of 1 teaspoon of activated charcoal dissolved in 1 cup of water, the blood is cleansed of toxins and impurities and the metabolic systems are supported for optimal fat digestion and processing of cholesterol. As a result, the heart and arteries receive the essential nutrients they need to achieve uninterrupted blood circulation to the entire body and brain. While activated charcoal should not be consumed in the same two-hour time span as other medications, the substance can be consumed safely at any other time throughout the day without any danger of side effects.

45: AIDS IN THE TREATMENT OF IRRITABLE BOWEL SYNDROME

Every year, an estimated 200,000 people suffer from irritable bowel syndrome (IBS). Not just an average everyday stomachache, IBS can develop such extremely painful symptoms that chronic sufferers experience serious interference in their everyday lives, sometimes being unable to socialize, work, or perform the most basic daily activities.

This chronic condition causes cramping, bloating, food intolerances, nausea, headaches, and interrupted bowel functions such as diarrhea or constipation. While heavy doses of antacids, anti-inflammatory drugs, and prescriptions promising enzymatic support are commonly prescribed, even the medical community is sometimes baffled by the persistence of the condition.

With the consumption of 1 teaspoon of activated charcoal dissolved in 1 cup of water daily, IBS sufferers can experience relief naturally and without any concern for harsh side effects that can aggravate their IBS or its associated symptoms. Activated charcoal has the ability to absorb and purge toxic substances and irritants from the body, but it's not only able to resolve inflammatory issues, toxicity, and infections that can contribute to disruptions leading to IBS flare-ups. It also helps the body's natural systems return to optimal functioning. Whether the digestive system needs support in producing acids and enzymes for proper digestion, the cardiovascular system requires a pathogens cleanse to prevent interference with metabolic processes, or hormonal balance needs restored after the onset of illness or disease, activated charcoal is able to remove harmful elements from affected systems and return the body to a normal, optimal, desirable way of functioning…naturally.

46: PROVIDES ANTIBACTERIAL PROTECTION

As you move through your average day, your exposure to bacteria is constant. On door handles, utensils, pens, surfaces, and in the air that flows around you, bacteria of countless forms thrive. If your immune system is healthy and your body's systems are functioning properly, these bacteria are simply processed and purged without any harm to the body and brain. If, however, the bombardment is severe enough or your immune system is compromised, the infiltration of bacteria can lead to serious health complications or even death.

While some types of bacteria are beneficial and play a positive role in the maintenance of certain functions and processes in the body, such as the digestion of foods and processing of nutrients, some other forms of bacteria are harmful and can wreak havoc on the body and mind. Affecting the skin, organs, and systems, harmful bacteria can contribute to the development of rashes and dermatitis, gastritis and ulcers, sexually transmitted diseases, and meningitis. When these conditions develop, the most readily prescribed treatments include antibiotics. But because antibiotics kill every kind of bacteria in your body, including the beneficial ones, the original disease can quickly return with exposure to the same bacteria, or new varieties can take advantage of your compromised system and cause new diseases.

With the ability to absorb and dispel microorganisms from the body and brain, consuming just 1 teaspoon of activated charcoal dissolved in 1 cup of water daily can offer effective prevention and treatment of bacterial infections. With the added benefit of natural immune system support, activated charcoal can help guard against consequential health conditions while promoting the body's naturally healthy functions.

47: PROVIDES ANTIMICROBIAL PROTECTION

The flu, Ebola, and various flesh-eating diseases are just a few of the frightening varieties of microbial infections that can lead to serious illness, disease, or even death. These harmful microbes are so powerful that they can change the body's chemical composition. When the chemical elements of the body are drastically altered, the rapid decline in health can decimate the immune system and allow microbes to infiltrate the body, divide and multiply, and wreak havoc on the organs and other functions.

Affecting everything from the skin, hair, and nails to the digestive system and brain, healthy and unhealthy microbial infiltration is ever-present.

Activated charcoal can flush destructive microbes from the body and is an all-natural approach to achieving overall health and wellness in almost every cell, organ, and system. Restoring the body's natural balance, activated charcoal helps the immune system defend against common infections and conditions, as well as hazardous microbes. By supporting other systems related to immunity, such as the digestive, cardiovascular, and nervous systems, activated charcoal helps the body perform like a well-oiled machine when it comes to preventing microbial illness and promoting optimal health and healing.

THE GOOD AND BAD OF MOTHER NATURE'S MICROBES

When most people think of microbes, the common misconception is that these "germs" cause harm. While there are countless microbes that can degrade health due to their consumption or "feeding on" nature's bounties of living organisms, there are health-improving microbes that benefit overall health too! With natural treatments like those that include activated charcoal, the toxic, harmful microbes that jeopardize health can be eliminated while the beneficial microbes that support health (through proceses like improving immunity or aiding digestion) can be safeguarded and supported safely.

48: BOOSTS ANTIFUNGAL PROTECTION

It's estimated that there are between 13,000 and 120,000 species of microfungi in the United States, and these microscopic organisms can thrive in damp, dark areas throughout the home and outside as well. While many varieties are harmless to humans, there are a number of microfungi that can adversely affect the body, causing infections every year.

With a healthy immune system providing protection against infection, the chances of a fungal infection spreading in or on the body can be minimized, but in any individual with a compromised immune system, the threat of fungal infection is very real. The most common infections related to microfungi affect the skin, lungs, blood, bones, tissues, and muscles, but they can also impact the nerves and brain. The most commonly diagnosed fungal infections include athlete's foot, jock itch, ringworm, and yeast infections, and these conditions are effectively treated with topical or oral antifungal medications. But while these treatments are often effective, activated charcoal can be used as a preventative and curative measure as well.

Activated charcoal can be used both as a topical treatment applied directly to the site of a fungal infection and as an oral application to purge the body of harmful pathogens. A solution of 1 teaspoon activated charcoal dissolved in 1 cup of water will expel internal fungal infections from the body's systems, helping boost immune system function and decrease healing time.

For topical treatments, a one-to-one ratio of activated charcoal and water or coconut oil can be applied directly to the site of the fungal infection, wrapped with a piece of gauze or fabric, and secured with surgical tape or plastic wrap. By employing both of these methods, recovery from a fungal infection can be achieved quickly, safely, and naturally.

49: HEALS SCALP CONDITIONS

Uncomfortable, unsightly, and embarrassing conditions that affect the scalp can ruin your day. From simple dandruff to excessive peeling and discoloration, scalp conditions can be acute or chronic and are almost always the result of one of the body's systems being out of balance. Without treatment, certain conditions can lead to serious scalp disorders that may even result in hair thinning or hair loss.

Many scalp conditions result from either a deficiency or a preexisting condition that causes the body's systems to function improperly. The most common scalp conditions are hair loss, head lice, male-pattern baldness, alopecia areata (hair loss in patchy areas), eczema, and psoriasis. In most cases, these conditions can be traced back to a chronic disease or disorder such as:

- Hashimoto's disease
- Hyperthyroidism
- Addison's disease
- Underactive pituitary gland
- Lupus
- Sclerosis
- Syphilis
- Celiac disease
- Malnutrition

A topical treatment that combines activated charcoal and water in a one-to-one ratio can be rubbed into the affected areas of the scalp for fifteen to sixty minutes three times a day, helping extract the unhealthy pathogens or organic compounds that have contributed to the scalp's affliction. In addition, ingesting 1 teaspoon of activated charcoal dissolved in 1 cup of water daily can help purge pathogens and toxins in the body that result in upsets to the immune system and compromised hormonal production. Naturally, and without the risk of side effects, activated charcoal can help resolve scalp conditions and contribute to healing within the body as well.

50: HELPS TREAT DIVERTICULITIS

More than 200,000 people are hospitalized with diverticulitis every year in America alone. This condition is caused by inflammation or infection in one of the folds or pockets of the digestive tract. When the small "pouches" found in the walls of the colon trap bits of undigested material, these settled organic compounds begin to rot and create a toxic reaction that leads to the development of inflammation. Once the body's inflammatory response sets in, the risk of infection skyrockets, and the result is a variety of physical ailments and symptoms, including:

- Fever
- Chills
- Bloating
- Gas
- Diarrhea
- Constipation
- Nausea
- Vomiting
- Loss of appetite
- Severe stomach pain (most commonly reported in the lower left side)
- Fatigue

These symptoms can last for a week or more if left untreated, so implementing preventative measures is key. By consuming a diet that includes plenty of fiber-rich foods, such as fruits and vegetables, the undigestible portions of foods join with acids in the stomach to produce a gel-like substance that sweeps away undigested bits of food and waste in the colon.

Consuming activated charcoal on a regular basis supports the digestive system too and removes toxic compounds that can contribute to infection and inflammation, the two most likely causes of diverticulitis flare-ups. A single teaspoon of activated charcoal dissolved in 1 cup of water taken daily can be an astoundingly effective preventative measure, and that same dosage can be consumed every few hours during times of diverticulitis upsets to minimize the painful symptoms and speed up healing naturally.

DIVERTICULITIS DIETARY RULES

Diverticulitis sufferers should avoid foods that can be easily trapped in the pockets that line the colon. These foods include nuts and seeds, such as sesame, sunflower, and poppy seeds. While seemingly safe, these tiny foods can contribute to diverticulitis by aggravating the uncomfortable symptoms that are commonly experienced during flare-ups.

PART 2

BEAUTY

It's estimated that the global beauty industry costs men and women around the world more than 100 billion dollars annually. Everyone everywhere is truly dedicated to their appearance, spending a combined 24 billion dollars on skin care products, 38 billion on hair care products, 18 billion on makeup, and 15 billion on perfume. These figures don't even include the services and treatments provided by physicians, specialists, and spas. While many beauty products that consumers buy promise to deliver results, many fail to meet their expectations. Even worse, because many beauty products contain synthetic additives and chemicals, some consumers experience complications and health disorders that can cause serious (and sometimes permanent) effects to their skin, hair, teeth, or overall body health.

Activated charcoal has proven to be an amazing ingredient in all areas of beauty, providing natural cleansing, exfoliation, and detoxification to the body. Whether your desire is to minimize wrinkles, fight acne, treat scalp and hair issues, or promote overall health through natural detoxification, activated charcoal can help. The entries in this section will provide recipes and instructions to help you create homemade soaps, creams, cleansers, and soaks that will not only help you achieve your beauty goals but also improve your overall health easily and naturally!

51: TREATS ACNE

Acne affects over 50 million Americans each year. The unsightly blemishes can appear seemingly out of nowhere, without cause, and can litter the face, back, shoulders, neck, and chest with irritating bumps, redness, and pus-filled pockets.

Acne is primarily caused by the buildup of oil and dead skin cells that blocks hair follicles. When these follicles are blocked, the glands that produce sebum, a natural oil that lubricates the hair and skin, are unable to secrete the substance, and the result is irritation, inflammation, and "whiteheads." Other contributing factors include elevated androgen and testosterone, hormonal fluctuations (as seen in puberty and pregnancy), menstruation, anxiety, stress, exposure to hot and humid clients, wearing oil-based makeup, and greasy hair.

With an all-natural two-step approach to healing acne that utilizes activated charcoal for internal and external healing, anyone can reduce the incidence of breakouts. First, for internal health, consume a simple teaspoon of activated charcoal dissolved in 1 cup of water up to three times daily to help purge the body's systems of toxins and pathogens that can interrupt immunity and hormonal functions, both of which can contribute to acne. Secondly, use the following activated charcoal body wash to help cleanse the skin.

TO MAKE A SIMPLE WASH FOR THE FACE OR BODY, USE:

1 part activated charcoal powder
1 part water

Combine the ingredients into a paste.

Apply to the afflicted areas and scrub to allow the charcoal to absorb and remove toxins, oils, and impurities that can interfere with normal follicle openings and the processes related to natural oil production at the skin's surface.

52: ALLEVIATES DANDRUFF

The common condition of dandruff can be embarrassing. While several over-the-counter products and prescription medications promise to provide relief, the underlying conditions often remain, allowing dandruff to persist after treatment. If you feel like your dandruff condition is unpredictable and always occurs unexpectedly, you'd probably be surprised to learn that even emotional disturbances can upset the balance of natural oils that help keep the scalp healthy. When there is an upset in your hormonal balance, hygiene regimen, or even stress and anxiety level, the scalp's dryness can develop the perfect conditions for the production of dandruff.

By using an activated charcoal treatment applied directly to the scalp, the conditions contributing to the development of dandruff can be resolved naturally. Eliminating toxins, regulating the pH balance of the skin, and removing environmental waste and hair care product residue from the scalp and hair are all ways that activated charcoal works to heal the scalp, returning the body to an optimally balanced hormonal condition and even killing the yeast that can play a major role in dandruff production.

TO MAKE AN ACTIVATED CHARCOAL HAIR RINSE, USE:

3 tablespoons activated charcoal powder

1 cup coconut oil

1 tablespoon lemon juice

Combine the ingredients in a jar and shake to mix thoroughly.

Apply the tonic to the scalp and leave on for 5–10 minutes before rinsing thoroughly.

RECOMMENDATIONS FOR USE:

If repeated daily, this simple application can rid the scalp of dryness and irritation naturally, without the harmful side effects of chemical-infused products that are normally applied to dandruff-ridden scalps.

Store remaining tonic in an airtight glass container with a tight-fitting lid. Keep the jar containing the tonic in a cool, dark place for 4–5 days.

53: WHITENS TEETH

Every year, an estimated 1.7 billion dollars are spent on teeth whitening pastes, treatments, and services. With all of the time and money spent seeking a brighter smile, an activated charcoal treatment may seem simplistic, but it can actually be effective, low in cost, and contribute added benefits to overall health. In numerous studies, activated charcoal has been compared to other popular teeth whitening processes and has proven to be the more effective solution.

A small amount applied to the teeth (1 opened capsule or crushed pressed pill, or a ¼ teaspoon of the fine powder alternative) unleashes activated charcoal's ability to adsorb and absorb toxins, organic compounds, and pathogens, ridding the mouth of the horrendous conditions that contribute to stained and yellow teeth.

Coffee, tea, wine, smoking, and consumption of unhealthy foods all contribute to the deposits of unhealthy discoloration on the teeth, but adopting a brushing regimen with a ¼ teaspoon of activated charcoal mixed with water that emulates normal brushing with toothpaste once or twice daily can help remove these stains. Using activated charcoal in this way also eliminates bacteria and pathogens from the mouth and protects teeth against the onset of decay.

THE SKINNY ON SENSITIVITY

While the desire to have whiter teeth is one that is shared among countless consumers around the world, the treatment methods used to achieve the aesthetically pleasing glowing smile can come at a serious cost: sensitivity. The caustic chemicals included in teeth whitening solutions can cause the stripping of enamel and the breakdown of protective elements of the teeth that prevent tingling and sensitivity to temperature, resulting in sensitivity. By opting for all-natural teeth-whitening methods such as those that include activated charcoal, apple cider vinegar, or coconut oil, anyone can achieve a whiter smile naturally and without the risks associated with synthetic solutions.

54: BALANCES OILY SKIN

Countless men and women struggle with oily skin, and they purchase hundreds of products and services that promise to provide protection against the condition that most often contributes to blemishes and breakouts. While poor hygiene is normally blamed for oily skin, there are a number of other causes, including:

1. Mental, emotional, or physical upsets
2. Overexertion and excessive exercise that leads to profuse sweating
3. Hormonal imbalances and fluctuations
4. A diet that includes excessive amounts of sugar-rich or fatty foods
5. Stress and anxiety

If you find yourself dealing with oily skin, even temporarily, there are a number of approaches you can take to regain a well-balanced complexion naturally. Avoiding harsh or abrasive chemical-laden products is imperative when dealing with oily skin because the underlying cause of excessive oil production can become even more aggravated by certain synthetic ingredients.

The use of activated charcoal—both internally and externally in simple, do-it-yourself combinations—can help anytime you feel your skin is out of balance. A capsule of activated charcoal combined with a small amount of water makes a refreshing moisturizer that can be applied gently to the entire face and then rinsed away. This helps the face by extracting toxins and harsh compounds, restoring a natural balance that helps reduce oil. You can also ingest 1 teaspoon of activated charcoal dissolved in 1 cup of water or an equivalent amount in pressed pill or capsule form of activated charcoal daily to gain optimal digestive, hormonal, and mental function, lending to overall skin health.

55: EXFOLIATES SKIN

Exfoliating the skin on the face and body is a highly recommended practice to keep it looking healthy and feeling refreshed. By removing dead cells on the skin's surface, exfoliation allows the skin to sweat, breathe, and purge toxins naturally. It also helps eliminate the dirt, grime, and natural by-products that can settle on the skin's surface and result in clogged pores and sweat glands. Regular exfoliation reduces acne and common blemishes naturally.

If you find yourself trying to determine the best exfoliant for your skin, the dizzying number of available products with their slew of questionable ingredients can make the search a little more difficult. Luckily there is an effective, all-natural approach to exfoliating your skin that you can make with a simple combination of healthy oils and activated charcoal.

Using an activated charcoal treatment exfoliates the skin, cleans dead skin cells, and even extracts toxins and compounds that can contribute to the development of skin issues. The coconut oil that's included in the following recipe is also a healthy, nourishing ingredient that can make the skin more supple over time.

TO MAKE AN EXFOLIATING SCRUB FOR THE FACE, USE:

1 tablespoon coconut oil
1–2 tablespoons activated charcoal powder

Combine the ingredients into a simple paste and apply it to the skin, gently massaging for 1–2 minutes before rinsing thoroughly.

TO MAKE AN EXFOLIATING SCRUB FOR THE WHOLE BODY, USE:

1 cup coconut oil
1–2 cups activated charcoal powder

Combine the ingredients into a paste and apply in the shower with circular massaging motions before rinsing away thoroughly.

56: MAKES AN ANTI-WRINKLE MASK

When the skin on the face is exposed to elements in the environment, it can develop a dull or aged appearance. Stress, anxiety, lack of sleep, smoking, and alcohol abuse can also contribute to the development of wrinkles. While pills and potions promise to reduce or eliminate wrinkles, these solutions rarely provide the results that wrinkle sufferers seek. To make the situation worse, some anti-wrinkle treatments, like Botox, can cause redness, inflammation, irritation, or paralysis of the face. But, with an all-natural approach to fighting wrinkles, you can support your skin's health and enjoy a glowing complexion without chemical-laden products.

By combining activated charcoal and a few other all-natural ingredients, you can create a cost-effective anti-wrinkle mask in your own home. The activated charcoal will extract toxins from the skin's surface and restore balance to oil-producing glands and the skin's pH. When you add in other healthy, antioxidant-rich ingredients like matcha powder, skin-soothing aloe vera, and moisturizing coconut oil, you will get a mask that maximizes your skin health while minimizing wrinkles.

TO MAKE THE MASK, COMBINE:

2½ teaspoons aloe vera

1 teaspoon witch hazel

2 teaspoons activated charcoal powder or 4600 mg of encapsulated or crushed pressed pill form

½ teaspoon matcha powder

2 teaspoons bentonite clay

2–5 drops tea tree oil

2–5 drops rosewood oil

6 drops eucalyptus oil

Combine all ingredients in a medium bowl and stir to mix thoroughly.

Apply an even layer of the mask to the face and allow to set for 20 minutes.

Rinse with warm water and apply a light application of a natural moisturizer.

RECOMMENDATIONS FOR USE:

For best results, this treatment should be repeated 2–3 times per week. Store mask mixture in a tightly sealed container and store in a cool, dry place for up to 2 weeks.

57: UNCLOGS PORES

Clogged pores can contribute to countless skin conditions, such as acne, blackheads, and a sluggish or lackluster complexion. Intent on having a complexion free of inflammation, irritation, and upset, many consumers desperately search to find products that will provide relief from clogged pores. To obtain that healthy skin glow, it is imperative that you purge the skin of toxins, impurities, and buildup that can contribute to blocked pores. When pores are blocked, they cannot receive the refreshing air, rejuvenating treatments, and cleansing regimens that allow the skin to breathe feely and feel and appear healthy. Many products and services that claim to unclog pores and remove impurities are invasive or contain additives that contribute to a "rebound effect," causing the pores to close up and become increasingly clogged as a result of their use.

You can make a simple at-home solution of activated charcoal and other all-natural ingredients that relieve toxicity, irritants, and inflammatory compounds. Activated charcoal's ability to adsorb, absorb, and extract toxins, impurities, chemical compounds, organic compounds, and environmental pollutants from the skin's pores helps restore a natural balance to oil production, dryness, and blemishes. It can even help combat wrinkles and discoloration caused by hormonal imbalances and pigmentation disruptions within the skin.

TO MAKE A PORE CLEANSING SOLUTION, USE:

1 tablespoon activated charcoal powder
1 tablespoon apple cider vinegar (unfiltered and organic)

Combine the two ingredients into a paste and apply to the skin of the face for 10–15 minutes before rinsing thoroughly. This application can be used daily or as often as needed throughout the week.

58: CLEANSES HAIR

Excessive product use, damaging styling regimens, consuming too many unhealthy foods, and even common health conditions can all contribute to buildup of excessive oils or residue resulting in hair that appears weighted down and greasy, or dry and brittle. Implementing a hair care regimen that naturally removes residue and buildup from everyday exposure to chemicals, toxins, environmental impurities, and pollution can help your hair regain a shiny, voluminous appearance and resume normal, optimal growth. While a quick look into any "clarifying" section of a hair care aisle makes obvious that plentiful products that aim to alleviate this issue are available, the concern is that harsh chemicals and additives included in these products can actually strip hair of essential oils and proteins that are required for hair health. The safer alternative to chemical-laden products that could cause more harm than good is one that includes an all-natural ingredient that removes buildup while safeguarding strands…such as treatments that include activated charcoal.

Adding a cleansing solution with activated charcoal into your weekly beauty routine can alleviate struggles with excessive buildup from toxicity, beauty supplies, and environmental pollution—all issues that contribute to weighted down hair.

TO CREATE A NATURAL HAIR CLEANSING RINSE, USE:

½ cup apple cider vinegar (organic and unfiltered)
1 tablespoon activated charcoal powder
1 cup water

Combine the ingredients in a container or bottle and shake vigorously to mix.

Apply the solution to your hair in the shower. Massage into the scalp and hair.

Let the application set for 3–5 minutes and then rinse thoroughly.

RECOMMENDATIONS FOR USE:

This rinse naturally rectifies unhealthy hair by extracting toxins, removing buildup, and absorbing toxins. While removing unhealthy elements, this treatment also safeguards the proteins and natural structures of hair strands naturally, so the treatment can be used safely as often as necessary. Apply as often as necessary until the hair returns to its desirable condition.

59: ADDS VOLUME TO HAIR

Almost every ad you see on television or in your favorite magazines promotes a product that promises to revitalize your hair so you can achieve that voluminous bounce and full, thick look everyone longs for. The countless hours spent in salons, applying products, teasing and treating our hair only seem to result in dull, dried out strands that become brittle and break. The underlying issue with these products is that the chemicals and additives that are added to the formulations can remove far more than just buildup; when applications that contain harsh abrasive components are applied to hair, the natural elements and processes that contribute to healthy hair strand composition and repair can be compromised, resulting in dry, frizzy, or unhealthy strands that are difficult to manage. In lieu of the synthetic products marketed to hopeful consumers seeking to add volume to their tresses, a do-it-yourself application can be made in your own kitchen using all-natural ingredients that not only add volume to hair but also a healthy shine and strength to every strand.

Activated charcoal has the ability to absorb and extract impurities, toxins, and harsh compounds from the scalp and hair, leaving them free of the elements that weigh hair down. Safely removing the toxic or harmful elements from the hair and scalp, activated charcoal is not only able to remove inhibiting elements but also promote proper production of proteins and support natural processes that contribute to hair health. When combined with organic apple cider vinegar that contains a protein-rich enzyme shown to repair and strengthen hair, the result is a head of voluminous tresses that didn't require the use of expensive, chemical-laden products.

TO MAKE A HAIR REPAIR RINSE, USE:

1 tablespoon activated charcoal powder

1 cup apple cider vinegar (organic, unpasteurized, and unfiltered)

1 tablespoon lemon juice

1 teaspoon coconut oil

Combine the ingredients (all at room temperature) in a jar and shake well until thoroughly combined.

Apply the solution to the hair and scalp while showering and leave in for 5 minutes.

Rinse your hair and style as normal. This application can be used 3 times weekly.

60: ACTS AS AN ANTI-AGING INGREDIENT

When people think of anti-aging products and services, the most common misconception is that they only apply to wrinkles and other aesthetic signs of natural aging. While wrinkles and various skin conditions can be obvious signs of aging, the true purpose of any anti-aging treatment is to defend against the corrosive, chemical-ridden and toxic attacks that can degrade the skin's cells and the cells that control the body's systems. By combining antioxidant-rich ingredients with activated charcoal, consumers seeking anti-aging benefits can achieve results easily at home without the risk of harsh side effects that are common among commercial anti-aging products and services.

"Turning back the clock" isn't simply about making the face and body appear younger. When you think of anti-aging, you should think about providing your entire body (including your cells, organs, and systems) with the health and rejuvenation it requires to function optimally. By supplementing the body with a natural healing element like activated charcoal, you can help your body purge harmful toxins and compounds from its cells and systems.

By combining two applications that utilize activated charcoal topically and internally, you can maximize the benefits even further. First, a topical application (such as the one presented in entry 56: Makes an Anti-Wrinkle Mask) can be used to heal and rejuvenate skin, making it appear less wrinkled, fatigued, and discolored with each passing day. Secondly, by consuming activated charcoal, the internal systems can benefit from the removal of waste and by-products acquired from food, water, and the environment. By ingesting just 1 teaspoon of activated charcoal dissolved in 1 cup of water daily, anyone seeking to reap the benefits of truly effective anti-aging can enjoy a gradual return to optimal health…from the inside and out.

61: MAKES A NATURAL EYELINER

An astounding number of eyeliners litter the shelves of every grocery and drugstore. Many claim to be hypoallergenic, all-natural, or organic, making it difficult to discern which product is the best choice. While these store-bought varieties may seem reputable, inexpensive, and easy, many of them can end up taking a toll on your wallet, your time, and your health. If you choose the wrong eyeliner that isn't appropriate for your skin or the condition of your eyes, the result can be irritation, inflammation, or infection that causes redness in and around the eyes, discharge, or even swelling. In order to avoid these undesirable and uncomfortable conditions, you can create your very own hypoallergenic eyeliner in the comfort of your own home using inexpensive, all-natural ingredients that support skin and eye health while highlighting the eyes in the same way as store-bought varieties.

Not only can you duplicate the aesthetic qualities of store-bought eyeliner, but you can also promote the health of your eyes and skin with the antibacterial, antiviral, and antimicrobial benefits of activated charcoal, as well as the moisturizing support of coconut oil. Reducing the risk of irritation, inflammation, and redness while also moisturizing the extremely sensitive skin around the eyes, this healthy, all-natural combination can be used as often as necessary.

TO CREATE A NATURAL EYELINER, USE:

1 teaspoon fine activated charcoal powder
1 tablespoon coconut oil

Combine both ingredients in a small glass jar with a tight-fitting lid and shake vigorously before every use.

RECOMMENDATIONS FOR USE:

A store-bought eyeliner applicator brush can be used to apply the solution around the eyes. Apply sparingly in order to achieve the desired effect. This application can be stored in any cool, dark area for up to 30 days.

62: CREATES A NATURAL MASCARA

For anyone who suffers from sensitive eye issues, such as inflammation, irritation, or redness, mascara can be a complicated purchase. Manufacturers and marketers involved in the production of mascara try to emphasize their products' ability to produce beautiful, lengthened, luxurious lashes with a simple swoop of a mascara brush. With the concern for eye health growing and eye sensitivity issues on the rise, mascara manufacturers have begun to focus on including "all-natural" ingredients that can help their products be more "eye-friendly." These hypoallergenic ingredients, however, are often far outweighed by synthetic ingredients, chemicals, dyes, and so on, leading to irritations, redness, and other adverse reactions.

In an effort to create a safer, truly all-natural, more health-promoting product that can achieve the same effect as store-bought mascaras, a number of consumers have turned to activated charcoal.

Helping to reduce the risk of allergic reactions, infections, inflammation, and redness, activated charcoal and coconut oil join forces in the following recipe to create the perfect alternative mascara for the consumer who desires an inexpensive, all-natural way to achieve long, luxurious lashes. Building better lashes and promoting overall health, this simple solution can make anyone love their lashes while safeguarding their eyes…naturally.

TO MAKE A CHARCOAL MASCARA, USE:

1 teaspoon fine activated charcoal powder
1 tablespoon coconut oil

Combine both ingredients in an emptied mascara tube and stir or shake the solution vigorously before use.

Apply to the lashes using the same method you would for a store-bought mascara, storing in any cool, dark area for up to 30 days.

63: FORMULATES A REJUVENATING FACE MASK

Whether you find yourself wishing that you could turn back the clock to restore your overall health and vigor or love how you feel and want your face to emulate your internal vitality, a rejuvenating face mask can help.

With a dizzying number of face masks filling the beauty aisle of almost every store imaginable, it can be hard to choose the right face mask for your skin type, your goals, and (most importantly) your sensitivities. Because many face masks contain harsh additives and chemicals that can deteriorate and degrade skin cells, an all-natural alternative is preferable to help detoxify the skin, repair its cells, and rejuvenate the entire face and neck.

Without the possibility of harmful side effects that can disrupt the appearance of the skin on the face and neck, a therapeutic mask derived from all-natural ingredients can be made quickly and inexpensively in the comfort of your own home. With activated charcoal starring in this DIY face mask, the health benefits go above and beyond simply rejuvenating the face.

TO CREATE YOUR OWN REJUVENATING FACE MASK, FOLLOW THESE STEPS:

¼ cup coconut oil
½ medium avocado
1 teaspoon activated charcoal
2 tablespoons lemon juice

In a blender, combine all ingredients and blend on high until thoroughly combined.

Apply mask to face and allow to set for 10–15 minutes.

Remove mask with a warm water rinse.

RECOMMENDATIONS FOR USE:

Utilize this treatment up to 3 times per week, discarding the remaining mask after each use.

64: CLEANSES SKIN

With the cleansing effect of soaps comes a common drying condition that can contribute to the cracking, irritation, and inflammation of the skin on the hands and body. If you find yourself searching for a healthy alternative to abrasive soaps that seem to remove dirt and grime effectively, this cleansing bar soap recipe will help you create your own varieties of organic bar soaps that not only cleanse but also purify and detoxify naturally.

By combining just a few healthy ingredients you may already have in your home, you can ditch the degrading bar soaps in your bathroom and atop your kitchen sinks. You can also add fragrance to these soaps with a number of scented natural oils, further enhancing the quality of these cleansing bars that will leave your skin feeling healthier than ever.

TO MAKE A CLEANSING RINSE, USE:

1 teaspoon activated charcoal powder
¼ cup lemon juice
¼ cup apple cider vinegar (organic, unpasteurized, and unfiltered)
1 cup Epsom salt
10 drops essential oil, such as lavender or sage (optional)

Combine all ingredients in a glass jar with a tight-fitting lid.

Shake jar or blend to combine all ingredients thoroughly.

Apply mixture to face and body, and massage gently for 15–30 seconds.

Rinse with warm water, followed by cold.

RECOMMENDATIONS FOR USE:

This mixture can be stored in a cool, dark place for up to 7 days. The treatment can be used daily or as often as desired.

65: EFFECTIVELY ELIMINATES BLACKHEADS

In the hustle and bustle of normal everyday life, the face and skin of the body can be exposed to countless toxins, pollutants, and organic and synthetic compounds that can pack the skin's pores with dirt and grime. Once the pores become polluted, clogs can lead to the development of blackheads on the face or body.

When the chemical compounds and synthetic additives found in manufactured soaps are applied to the skin's surface, the pores can become agitated and can develop further blemishes besides blackheads, including acne, whiteheads, discoloration, redness, inflammation, and irritation.

By utilizing a combination of activated charcoal and a soothing, fragrance-free moisturizer, natural oil, or simple water, you can create a cleansing application that detoxifies the pores from pollutants, allowing them to breathe, and return the skin's surface back to optimal health. With the added benefits of additional ingredients that help absorb moisture, anyone can prevent blackheads and unsightly or unhealthy skin conditions quickly, easily, and naturally.

TO CREATE AN AT-HOME BLACKHEAD-SOLVING SOLUTION, FOLLOW THIS RECIPE:

1 ½ teaspoons bentonite clay

1 teaspoon activated charcoal powder

1 teaspoon apple cider vinegar (organic and unfiltered)

1 ½ tablespoons coconut oil

Combine all ingredients in a bowl and whisk together thoroughly.

Apply to the face generously in circular motions.

Leave treatment on the site of application for 15–20 minutes.

Remove using warm water on a moist towelette.

Moisturize as usual.

RECOMMENDATIONS FOR USE:

This application can also be used on other areas of the body that are affected by blackheads by following the same instructions for application. The treatment can be stored in an airtight glass container in a cool, dark place for 5–7 days.

66: CLARIFIES HAIR

A number of products on the market claim to clarify hair riddled with buildup from products, services, and treatments over time. Daily exposure to environmental pollutants, toxins, organic and inorganic compounds, unhealthy bacteria, microfungi, and algae that can be carried on every gust of wind also contribute to the buildup that can make hair feel weighed down, frizzy, or adversely reactive to normal hair care regimens.

In many "clarifying" hair care products, the ingredients can include astringents and alcohols that not only remove dirt and grime but also complicate the natural protein-rich strength of hair, causing damage to hair follicles at their root. All of these complications can create conditions that irritate the scalp, hinder the hair's natural growth, and inhibit the systematic processes that support hair's healthy appearance.

With a simple, inexpensive clarifying solution that you can make easily in your home, you can rely on the detoxifying and purifying properties of activated charcoal to remove excessive buildup from hair and purge toxicity and environmental compounds. This hair rinse recipe also uses organic apple cider vinegar for its all-natural enzymes that can contribute to the protein-related processes that are necessary to achieving healthy hair.

TO MAKE A CLARIFYING HAIR RINSE, USE:

1 cup apple cider vinegar (organic and unfiltered)
2 tablespoons of activated charcoal powder

Combine both ingredients in a glass jar and shake to dissolve the charcoal.

Apply to hair in the shower and let set for 5 minutes.

Rinse thoroughly. When the process is completed, you can dry and style hair as usual.

RECOMMENDATIONS FOR USE:

Use the treatment as often as necessary, and store any remaining solution in a cool, dark place for up to 1 week.

67: MAKES A CLEANSING BODY SCRUB

With countless brands promoting their body scrubs as the most refreshing, rejuvenating, or revitalizing option, it can be somewhat surprising to realize that many contain harsh ingredients that can actually dry out the skin and contribute to acne, irritation, inflammation, and eczema. Even products that promote themselves as "all-natural" normally contain ingredients that are synthetic additives or preservatives that risk irritating the skin or clogging pores.

While these cleverly marketed cleansing scrubs are presented in appealing packaging, use attractive buzzwords, and claim to provide the skin with relief and restoration, buyers should know that an all-natural alternative can be made easily in your home and for a low cost. You can create your very own activated charcoal–based body scrub (with no concern for harmful side effects) that contains a healthy combination of skin-soothing ingredients and can be used as often as necessary to relieve skin issues or restore vitality.

Activated charcoal's ability to detoxify the skin of harmful chemicals and compounds is accompanied by soothing aloe that not only relieves skin irritations but also contributes to the healthy regeneration of skin cells. The addition of moisturizing coconut oil helps this unique scrub promote moisture retention in the skin for hours after its use.

TO CREATE THIS AT-HOME ACTIVATED CHARCOAL RECIPE, USE:

1 teaspoon activated charcoal powder

1 cup brown sugar

½ cup coconut oil

¼ cup grapefruit juice

10 drops essential oils such as lavender or sage

In a glass jar with a tight-fitting lid, combine all ingredients and stir to combine thoroughly.

Apply generous amounts of the cleansing treatment to the skin's surface and massage gently.

Rinse with warm water and moisturize.

RECOMMENDATIONS FOR USE:

Use daily and store in a cool, dry place.

68: CREATES A NATURAL EYEBROW GEL

With age and the onset of numerous illnesses, conditions, and diseases that can wreak havoc on the skin and hair, the eyebrows become a proverbial "window to the soul" that can either indicate vitality or a lack thereof. Of the many new cosmetic procedures intended to bring a sense of youthfulness back to the skin, face, neck, eyes, and mouth, the most surprising may be services promising to bring a youthful look back to the eyebrows.

Brands from all over the world have recognized the new need for eyebrow-enhancing products that make the eyes "pop" and have responded with an overwhelming number of products and services. Eyebrow threading, eyebrow lifts, and permanent brow shading, among others, are becoming more and more popular in spas, salons, and even shopping malls, but this new approach to fuller, more luxurious-looking eyebrows can be quite costly.

You can make an eyebrow gel in your own home for a fraction of the price and without concern for any skin issues that could result from the use of harsh ingredients that some over-the-counter beauty products contain.

TO CREATE YOUR OWN EYEBROW GEL FORMULATION, SIMPLY FOLLOW THESE STEPS:

1 tablespoon aloe vera gel

½ teaspoon activated charcoal powder

In a small glass container with a tight-fitting lid, pour aloe vera gel and gradually mix in activated charcoal until desired tint is achieved.

Apply gel to eyebrows with a small makeup brush and smooth and shape until desired effect is achieved.

RECOMMENDATIONS FOR USE:

The mixture can be stored in a cool, dark area for up to 30 days. Apply as often as necessary to achieve and maintain desired look.

69: REMOVE TOXINS WITH A BATH SOAK

When the stress of everyday life ends up wearing you out and weighing you down, it can be nice to relax in a calming bath. If you find yourself stressed, anxious, overwhelmed, irritable, sick with a cold or flu, or battling an injury or disease, one of the best things you can do for your body is to rest and relax in a detoxifying bath soak.

Helping to withdraw impurities, toxins, and unhealthy organic and inorganic compounds from the body, activated charcoal can work wonders to return your body to a healthy state without the irritation and inflammation that can occur from store-bought, synthetic products.

This make-it-yourself combination of simple ingredients is an all-natural approach to an inexpensive detox soak that can be used as often as necessary without concern for harsh chemicals, synthetic additives, or overexposure.

TO MAKE THE SOAK, SIMPLY FOLLOW THIS RECIPE:

4 cups Epsom salt
⅛ cup activated charcoal powder
½ cup coconut oil
½ cup aloe vera
25 drops scented essential oil (optional)

Pour all ingredients at the water flow point on the floor of a bathtub and draw a bath with warm to hot water that is able to be tolerated for 15–20 minutes.

Submerge the entire body in the water and relax for 15–20 minutes.

Drain the tub, rinsing the sides of the remnant ingredients.

Shower off using temperate water and dry off as usual.

RECOMMENDATIONS FOR USE:

This treatment can be used as often as 5 times per week and for as long as 30 minutes.

70: TREATS BURNS

When the skin's surface is burned, the body reacts in a very protective way. Sending a surge of white blood cells to immediately fend off any possible infection, the body begins the reparative process for regenerating the skin and restoring the health of remaining skin cells. Because burns can affect multiple layers of the skin, burn categories have been used to identify, describe, and determine the amount of damage associated with each type of burn. Not only does this help with diagnosing burns and the common conditions associated with each type, but it also helps in the determination of the most effective treatment method to use.

Because burns have such a high risk of infection, it is imperative to use antibacterial, antiviral, and antimicrobial agents immediately following the burn incident and throughout the treatment process as well. Activated charcoal helps prevent bacteria, viruses, and microbes from infecting burn wounds and aids in extracting toxins, impurities, and even lingering carcinogenic bits from burned skin. When combined with soothing aloe that has been shown to work wonders with burns, activated charcoal is able to transcend deeper into the layers of the skin and help the body's repair process move more quickly. With aloe's ability to provide plentiful antioxidants, analgesic compounds for pain, and nutrients, the combination of these two ingredients has shown great success as an all-natural approach to healing burns.

TO MAKE A TOPICAL SOLUTION TO HEAL BURNS, USE:

1 teaspoon activated charcoal
3–4 tablespoons aloe vera

Combine the two ingredients and apply the mixture to the site of a burn. Wrap in gauze, and then secure it with a bandage, tape, or even plastic wrap to seal the application in tightly.

RECOMMENDATIONS FOR USE:

The application can be applied as often as necessary and should be used until the burn has fully healed. Remaining treatment should be stored in an airtight glass container in a cool, dark place for 5–7 days.

71: REJUVENATES SKIN WITH A CHARCOAL–LEMON JUICE MASK

Lemon juice has some pretty amazing qualities that can help facial skin in countless ways. Rich in vitamin C, lemon juice–based masks and toners have become increasingly popular among those who hope to save their skin from aging, sun damage, environmental pollution, toxicity, or buildup from skin care products. Many people are surprised to discover that lemon juice can even help minimize the irritation and inflammation that's commonly associated with redness, itchiness, blotches, and hyper- or hypopigmentation.

With the addition of activated charcoal, lemon juice–based applications can improve and protect the health of skin even more. While store-bought applications (even those claiming to be all-natural or organic) promise to deliver results, many can have harsh additives and ingredients that actually exaggerate facial skin issues or exacerbate underlying conditions. Pills, potions, and rinses that aren't made at home with all-natural ingredients will always come with the risk of side effects. Keeping that in mind, most people who find out how simple and easy it is to make your very own mask treatment from activated charcoal and lemon juice find it to be an optimal alternative.

TO MAKE THE FACE MASK, USE:

2 tablespoons lemon juice
4 tablespoons mashed avocado
1 teaspoon activated charcoal powder

Combine the ingredients in a bowl.

Apply the mask directly to the face and allow to set for 5–10 minutes before rinsing.

RECOMMENDATIONS FOR USE:

You can use this mask up to 3 times a week and refrigerate the remaining mask mixture in an airtight container after each use.

72: MAKES A NATURAL FACIAL CLEANSER

With the skin on certain areas of the body requiring more sensitive attention than others, it can be difficult to maintain a skin care regimen that addresses each area of need individually with the appropriate cleansers. The skin on the arms and legs requires much less sensitive ingredients than the areas of the chest, shoulders, and back, just as the face requires a far more sensitive application.

There are still certain conditions, such as acne and blackheads, that can make the use of harsher, "more effective" cleansers seem appealing. However, products that contain strong astringents, acids, and compounds actively strip the skin, erode certain elements, and purge the pores, leaving skin dry, irritated, and inflamed.

With an all-natural approach to facial cleansing, the ingredients you may have right in your own home can play a major role in restoring your skin's natural balance and minimizing common conditions…without the risk of serious side effects.

Activated charcoal can be incorporated into a simple face wash solution that extracts toxins, restores pH balance, controls oil, and removes dirt and grime, in addition to minimizing the effects that irritants and inflammatory compounds have created.

TO MAKE AN ACTIVATED CHARCOAL FACE WASH, FOLLOW THESE STEPS:

¼ cup coconut oil

⅛ cup aloe vera

2 teaspoons activated charcoal

2 tablespoons lemon juice

1 tablespoon grapeseed oil

In a blender, combine all ingredients and blend on high until mixed thoroughly.

Apply treatment to face and massage with fingertips for 15–30 seconds.

Rinse face with warm or cold water and towel dry.

Moisturize as necessary.

RECOMMENDATIONS FOR USE:

This treatment can be stored in an airtight glass container with a tight-fitting lid in a cool dark area for 5–7 days. Use as often as once per day.

73: REPAIRS FACIAL HEALTH WITH A TURMERIC AND CHARCOAL MASK

The ingredients in this mask can help you obtain a healthy overall glow, providing reparative benefits that continue to heal, protect, and moisturize long after it's been rinsed away.

With turmeric's amazing ability to apply countless antioxidants and anti-inflammatory compounds to the skin, this combination of all-natural ingredients is not only ideal for the face but also any irritated area that requires effective and immediate relief.

Because aloe has the ability to speed the healing process, this mask is able to penetrate deeply into subdermal layers of the skin, delivering the potent antioxidants and anti-inflammatory compounds to the cells beneath the surface.

The activated charcoal in this mask helps remove impurities and toxins, restore an optimal balance of oils, and clear pores of clogs and pollutants. As an added bonus, the addition of coconut oil provides extra moisture.

Combine the turmeric, coconut oil, and aloe in a bowl and whisk thoroughly.

Slowly add in the charcoal. As a paste develops, you will notice the thickness and color change, indicating the complete binding of all ingredients.

Once the paste thickens, apply to the face immediately and allow to set for 10 minutes before rinsing thoroughly.

RECOMMENDATIONS FOR USE:

This application can be used daily or as needed and should be stored in an airtight container at room temperature in a dry place for up to 1 week. Do not place the mixture in the refrigerator as this will cause the coconut oil to coagulate.

TO CREATE THIS MASK, USE:

1 teaspoon turmeric
2 tablespoons coconut oil
2 tablespoons aloe
1 teaspoon activated charcoal powder

74: HEALS CRACKED LIPS

The condition of chapped lips is one of the most aggravating to deal with because it can be challenging to resolve. With an overabundance of environmental factors, illnesses, and lifestyle habits that can contribute to the development of chapped lips, it's no surprise that countless Americans suffer from the condition multiple times throughout the year. Whether the root cause is cold air, smoking, drinking excessive amounts of alcohol, dry mouth, dehydration, or repeated exposure to saliva, chapped lips can cause pain, redness, irritation, swelling, cracking, and even infection.

Over-the-counter chap-relieving sticks and balms promise to provide relief, but the sensitive skin of the lips can react adversely to chemicals, synthetic additives, bacteria, and microorganisms present within these solutions. In an effort to combat these issues, many people opt for pricier varieties of lip-soothing applications that advertise the use of organic or all-natural ingredients, but this clever marketing strategy can actually mask the inclusion of harsh additives and preservatives used to prolong shelf life.

The following recipe is a truly all-natural combination of organic ingredients you can source at home to create a soothing chapped-lip reliever that can be kept in your pocket, purse, or car for use anytime you feel dry, chapped conditions developing on your lips. Use of this treatment at the first sign of chapping is highly recommended in order to prevent your lips from getting worse or possibly getting infected.

TO MAKE THE CHAPPED LIP TREATMENT, FOLLOW THESE STEPS:

3 teaspoons natural, organic, unbleached beeswax
5 teaspoons jojoba or coconut oil
¼ teaspoon activated charcoal
1 teaspoon honey
8 drops essential oil of your choice

Add beeswax and oil to a glass bowl and place in the microwave on high for 45–60 seconds to melt.

Mix in the activated charcoal, honey, and essential oil and mix until thoroughly combined.

Pour the mixture into small glass containers with tight-fitting lids, and leave uncovered until cooled.

RECOMMENDATIONS FOR USE:

Store in a cool, dark area for regular use whenever desired for up to 30 days.

75: PROMOTES HEALING OF COLD SORES

As unsightly and uncomfortable as cold sores may seem, their underlying cause can make anyone's stomach turn. Bacteria, viruses, and microbes can sit in the corners of the mouth, breeding until the infestation breaks into the skin and develops an obvious sore. Whether the underlying cause is internal or external, the resulting sore on the lips can be an open wound that will continue to worsen over time from exposure to countless germs caused by saliva and certain foods, drinks, and toxins that can irritate the skin.

By using a two-step approach to combat cold sores, anyone suffering from prolonged or acute cold sores can prevent their development and speed up the healing time of those that do appear. With the simple ingestion of activated charcoal daily, the body is able to purge the harsh bacteria, viruses, and microbes that can contribute to cold sore development. When the organic and inorganic elements that cause this condition are unable to breed, the result is an improved immune system that is able to combat illness more efficiently.

In addition to the ingestion of activated charcoal, the topical applications of lip balms (please see the following entry) containing activated charcoal can also help reduce the incidence of cold sore development and contribute to healing the existing conditions that contribute to their growth and persistence.

76: MAKES A NATURAL LIP BALM

Countless lip balms are sold every year, promising to provide rejuvenation to lips. With the plethora of products available, it can be easy to fall victim to marketing ploys that advertise long-lasting moisture, medicinal relief, or appealing colors, scents, and flavors. While these creative ads and promotions may make a product seem worth the price, hidden dangers and health risks lurk behind the persuasive packaging.

Many lip balms use synthetic ingredients, harsh additives, preservatives, and even some ingredients that cause serious harm to the environment. Palm oil is one of the most common lip balm ingredients, and its harvesting is ravaging certain areas of the Earth by eliminating a natural resource that plays a major role in the ecosystem.

A truly all-natural lip balm can be created at home using organic ingredients found in your own cupboard, providing relief from chapping, protection against infection, and a beautiful sheen that looks great and tastes great too!

TO MAKE THIS NATURAL LIP BALM, USE:

2 tablespoons beeswax pellets

2 tablespoons shea butter

2 tablespoons coconut oil

¼ teaspoon activated charcoal powder

15 drops essential oil (optional)

Combine all ingredients in a small pot over medium heat.

When all ingredients are melted and thoroughly combined (about 5 minutes), remove from heat.

Pour cooled (but not coagulated) lip balm into an airtight container with a tight-fitting lid.

RECOMMENDATIONS FOR USE:

Apply balm to lips as often as necessary, when irritation, discomfort, or dryness presents itself. The balm should be stored in cool, dark areas and can be used regularly for 30 days.

77: PROMOTES NUTRIENT ABSORPTION

A little-known fact about the development of chronic conditions (everything from fatigue to diabetes to obesity) is that they can all stem from one thing: the inability to process essential nutrients properly. People across the globe suffer from chronic and acute medical conditions that can affect any cell, organ, or system, wreaking havoc on everyday life.

Pharmaceutical companies do their best to promote their medications for almost every imaginable condition, but the treatments they provide are just that: treatments. Simply treating the symptoms of a disease may provide relief temporarily, but it rarely cures the underlying condition that causes the symptoms. Preventative treatments address the actual cause of an illness or disease, allowing existing symptoms to subside and keeping new ones from occurring by boosting the body's immune response.

Activated charcoal can benefit the body in countless ways, but namely by absorbing the toxins, impurities, and compounds that commonly interfere with proper nutrient absorption. When activated charcoal absorbs and extracts interfering elements from the body's cells, organs, and systems, the body is able to function as intended.

A simple teaspoon of activated charcoal dissolved in water and consumed daily can help anyone improve their body's ability to process nutrients, maintain the health of their body's systems, and safeguard their immune system and cells from degradation and complications. Supporting everything from heart health to brain health to hormone production, anyone's well-being and vitality can be simply and easily restored...naturally.

78: MOISTURIZES SKIN

Skin that feels dry and in need of moisture can quickly snowball into a majorly uncomfortable, or even seriously dangerous, condition. While most people moisturize their skin for aesthetic reasons or to alleviate the mild discomfort of dry skin, some people suffer from seriously dry patches of skin that can be isolated to one or more areas—even the entire body. Those who suffer from chronically dry skin can develop cracking and wounds that require medical attention or risk the possibility of infection.

Whether the goal is to spot-treat certain areas or soothe a severe bout of dry skin, a moisturizer that includes activated charcoal, aloe vera, and shea butter can provide long-lasting moisture that meets or exceeds what's offered by over-the-counter products.

Aloe has been used for centuries to provide penetrating, soothing relief to skin irritations and inflammation. The aloe and shea butter pair nicely to provide preventative protection in addition to immune system support and skin cell health. Activated charcoal acts as a detoxification aid, removing the impurities of the skin that can cause dryness.

TO MAKE THIS MOISTURIZER, USE:

2 teaspoons activated charcoal powder

2 tablespoons aloe vera

1 cup shea butter

1–2 drops lavender, eucalyptus, or other essential oil (optional)

Whisk the charcoal and the aloe vera until thoroughly combined.

Place the shea butter in a jar and add the aloe and activated charcoal mixture, combining thoroughly.

If you'd like to add fragrance, add a few drops of your preferred oil gradually until all ingredients are thoroughly combined.

RECOMMENDATIONS FOR USE:

This moisturizer can be applied as often as necessary for relief from dryness, discomfort, or skin irritation. The moisturizer should be stored in an airtight glass container in a cool, dark area for up to 30 days.

79: PROMOTES HAIR GROWTH

The desire to grow thick, lengthy hair is one shared by countless people around the world. Bombarded by messages that beauty is defined by the aesthetically pleasing appearance of elegant tresses, this goal is not unfounded. With the demand being high, the beauty industry has responded with countless hair growth products and services that range in price from just a few dollars to hundreds or even thousands. Promising to provide the stimulation and nutrition that's necessary for optimal hair growth, these products often fail to deliver those results.

A number of physicians, medical professionals, and natural health practitioners have spoken out against the use of these products because of their dangerous inclusion of harsh chemicals and additives that can do serious damage to the body. Because they are applied directly to the sensitive follicles that line the thin skin of the scalp, these products' ingredients are absorbed through the skin and can travel directly into the bloodstream and throughout the body. The toxins and impurities that these chemicals deliver to the brain and body can be disastrous to one's health.

Consuming just 1 teaspoon of activated charcoal dissolved in 1 cup of water daily will help remove toxins and impurities that can interfere with the circulatory system, hormone production, and metabolic processes, all of which directly affect hair growth. As an added benefit, activated charcoal can be used in a number of hair care applications that cleanse the hair of impurities (see entry 58), remove residue (see entry 52), and open the hair follicles to protein absorption and processing for longer, stronger, thicker hair!

80: MAKES DIY PORE STRIPS

The appearance of large pores on the face can occur for a number of reasons, including malnutrition, dehydration, or illness. For many, a simple detoxification process can help minimize the size and appearance of pores. Returning pores to a healthy, cleansed state that results in a softer, more luminous appearance, this detoxifying pore application is similar to the pore strips and peels that are available at your favorite grocery or drugstore. However, unlike store-bought products, this application relies on activated charcoal to intensify the detoxification results naturally.

Manufactured pore strips use glues, adhesives, and harsh chemicals that can tear away healthy skin cells along with blackheads and dead skin cells, making skin irritation a real risk for consumers of these products. In contrast, this DIY pore refining mask uses gelatin as a bonding agent, ensuring that anyone can gently apply and peel away the treatment without harming healthy skin and causing inflammation and irritation. With the added benefit of activated charcoal to remove impurities and toxins, the manufactured alternatives can't even compare.

TO MAKE THIS MASK, YOU WILL NEED:

1 tablespoon gelatin
1 teaspoon activated charcoal powder
2 tablespoons organic milk
Applicator stick (for applying mask)

In a microwave-safe glass bowl, combine gelatin, charcoal, and milk and stir until creamy.

Microwave on high for 15 seconds and allow to cool about 30 seconds, or until it can be applied without burning the skin.

Use applicator stick to apply generously to the face. Allow to set for 15 minutes and then peel off.

Moisturize after 30–60 minutes.

RECOMMENDATIONS FOR USE:

Leftover pore strip solution can be stored in an airtight glass container in a cool, dark area for up to 7 days.

81: REMOVES MAKEUP NATURALLY

Removing "long-lasting" or waterproof makeup can be challenging, and the beauty industry has responded with a number of products that promise to safely remove even the most stubborn makeup. While these products sometimes tout their "natural" ingredients, a high percentage of them actually contain ingredients that can irritate the sensitive skin of the face and lips and cause major upset to the eyes.

Your best bet for makeup removal that's free of side effects is to create your very own at-home application using all-natural ingredients like activated charcoal. Inexpensive and packed with benefits, this makeup remover can cleanse your face while also providing detoxification and protection against damage.

TO CREATE A NATURAL MAKEUP REMOVER, FOLLOW THESE STEPS:

4 tablespoons coconut oil
2 cups water
1 tablespoon activated charcoal powder

In a microwave-safe bowl, combine the coconut oil and water and microwave on high for 15–30 seconds, or until the coconut oil is softened or melted.

Whisk in the activated charcoal powder until thoroughly combined.

Pour the mixture into a glass or plastic container that can be sealed completely.

Shake bottle well before each use. To remove makeup, apply solution to a cotton ball or paper towel.

Gently massage the solution onto the skin until all makeup has been removed.

Rinse face completely.

RECOMMENDATIONS FOR USE:

The solution should be stored in an airtight glass container in a cool, dark area for up to 30 days.

HARMFUL INGREDIENTS ARE EVERYWHERE

In an unassuming product like makeup remover, the ingredients can seem harmless, but a consumer has to consider what's chemically required to make these products so effective at removing waterproof or smudge-proof makeup. Activated charcoal, on the other hand, doesn't contain any harsh ingredients or have any side effects, and anyone can use it in conjunction with simple, natural oils or aloe to match the results of almost any commercially available beauty product.

82: PREVENTS SKIN INFECTIONS

The surface of the skin is intended to protect against the infiltration of harmful pathogens, and it does this best when it's not afflicted with a compromising condition. When the skin is compromised, even a slight infection has the potential to develop into a serious illness that can plague the blood, cells, organs, and systems without warning. By taking the necessary measures to address skin issues quickly and properly, you can ensure that a simple skin condition doesn't progress into something more.

Using activated charcoal to make your own topical skin infection treatment eliminates the need to expose your vulnerable skin to the kinds of unnatural ingredients found in standard treatments. The activated charcoal in the following recipe acts swiftly to attract and absorb toxins and impurities while soothing aloe vera penetrates deep into numerous layers of the skin. This dual-action process has a detoxifying effect on wounds, providing protection against pathogens and acting as an analgesic for pain and inflammation at or beneath the skin's surface.

TO MAKE A TOPICAL SKIN TREATMENT, USE:

2 tablespoons activated charcoal powder
2 tablespoons aloe vera

Combine the ingredients into a paste and apply to the site of concern. Wrap with a paper towel or gauze and secure the wrap with a bandage or plastic wrap for up to 4 hours, allowing the ingredients to work hand-in-hand to effectively remove harmful compounds.

PEROXIDE: THE WORST APPLICATION FOR SKIN IRRITATIONS

Though peroxide has long been used to treat infections, irritations, and even cuts and burns, scientists have demonstrated in numerous studies that this commonly used treatment can actually harm skin cells and inhibit their repair. Instead of peroxide solutions, applications using moisturizing ingredients such as aloe and natural oils, in combination with activated charcoal, are a more effective way to heal and repair harmed cells.

83: MAKES AN EVENING FACIAL MOISTURIZER

The face is exposed to a constant barrage of irritants throughout the day, and nighttime is the perfect opportunity to provide your skin with restorative and reparative relief.

You can formulate your own moisturizer with the help of a simple recipe that you can customize to your skin's needs. You can also add certain oils, juices, or even fragrances to further enhance your moisturizer according to your preferences.

Apply 1 teaspoon of the mixture to the palm of the hand and, using the fingertips of the opposite hand, apply the moisturizer to the face in small amounts, swirling slowly in circular motions.

Allow the moisturizer to set and absorb before sleeping.

In the morning, rinse thoroughly and apply makeup or routine beauty applications as normal.

TO MAKE THIS NIGHTTIME MOISTURIZER, USE:

1 cup coconut oil
¼ teaspoon fine activated charcoal powder
½ teaspoon vitamin E
¼ teaspoon essential oil of your choice (optional)

*Additions for specific conditions: Choose one according to skin type/need:
1 teaspoon lemon juice (oily skin)
1 teaspoon shea butter (dry skin)
1 teaspoon grapeseed oil (wrinkled skin)
1 teaspoon aloe vera (irritated or inflamed skin)

In a glass jar with a tight-fitting lid, combine ingredients and use an immersion blender to mix thoroughly.

RECOMMENDATIONS FOR USE:

Moisturizer should be stored in an airtight glass container in a cool, dark place for up to 30 days.

SKIN TYPE MATTERS

When choosing your perfect facial moisturizer, your skin type matters. For those who suffer from oily or greasy skin, moisturizers that contain butters or oils can contribute to the development of acne. Overly dry skin conditions can be made worse with alcohol-based ingredients. If you don't remain aware of the type of skin you're treating, your skin improvement efforts could be counterproductive.

84: MINIMIZES FACIAL ACNE

While unsightly blemishes are what most people think of when they hear the word *acne*, the fact of the matter is that acne can occur at any subdermal layer of the skin creating cysts, irritation, or whiteheads without warning. Underlying conditions such as stress, hormonal imbalance, exposure to pesticides or pathogens, malnutrition (or the inability to absorb and process nutrients properly), chronic illnesses, and even tight-fitting clothes can all contribute to the development of unsightly facial acne.

When the skin is exposed to pollutants, internal toxicity, and stresses that interfere with normal systematic functions each and every day, it can be difficult to keep body acne in check. The daily implementation of a topical application that cleanses and detoxifies the skin's surface, in conjunction with an all-natural oral supplement that absorbs and extracts toxins, can help anyone find natural relief from acne.

Whether it's acute or chronic, isolated to one area or prevalent all over the face, acne can be naturally relieved without the need for prescription or over-the-counter medications, special shampoos and cleansers, or fortified soaps and salves. A simple two-step approach to treating the internal conditions that contribute to acne and its external symptoms will help body acne dissipate and prevent future outbreaks.

The simple addition of 1 teaspoon of activated charcoal daily to food or drinks can combat and prevent infections that compromise immunity and interrupt natural system functions that are related to skin health. Externally, the body scrub in entry 67 and the calming bath soak in entry 69 are also appropriate for everyday use.

85: SOOTHES SUNBURNS

Exposure to sunlight can lead to sunburns. While the symptoms of this skin condition may seem limited to aggravation or simple discomfort, the skin can sometimes blister and peel as a result, leaving it vulnerable to infections by bacteria, viruses, and microbes that can lurk anywhere.

The true dangers of sunburns lie beneath the skin, hidden from the naked eye. When sunburns set in, the skin cells that are damaged can become cancerous, leading to carcinogenic mutations. Not only are the specific skin cells of the sunburned region adversely affected, but these cellular mutations can actually lead to the cancerous mutations of other cells throughout the body, otherwise known as "metastasization." When this occurs, the cancerous cells are able to flow freely throughout the bloodstream and body, wreaking havoc on healthy cells.

In an effort to minimize the negative effects of sunburns, it is highly recommended that anyone who anticipates prolonged sun exposure wear protective sunscreen, clothing, hats, and eyewear. If a sunburn does develop, you can use a topical solution of activated charcoal and aloe to provide topical pain relief and help protect the cells from free radical damage that can cause cancerous mutations. Ingesting 1 teaspoon of activated charcoal dissolved in 1 cup of water daily is another way to combat free radical damage, toxicity, and immune system malfunctions that can all contribute to the development of harmful conditions in individuals with a history of excessive sunburns.

TO MAKE THIS SKIN-SOOTHING GEL, USE:

1 teaspoon activated charcoal powder
½ cup aloe vera

Mix the ingredients together. Apply to affected areas and cover with clothing. (Be ready to discard the clothing after use.) Use as often as necessary for relief. This treatment can be stored in an airtight glass container in a cool, dark area for up to 30 days.

86: MINIMIZES AGE SPOTS

Age spots, also referred to as "liver spots," are unsightly areas of hyper- or hypopigmentation that can result from prolonged sun exposure, previous skin issues, and even illnesses and disease. Age spots can be an indicator of past or present health conditions.

A number of prescriptions and over-the-counter products promise to minimize the appearance of age spots, but these products often contain harsh chemicals that can bleach the skin of pigment in the areas they're applied, contribute to irritation and inflammation, or even worsen the appearance by highlighting areas of hyper- or hypopigmentation. In an effort to fight the appearance of age spots without the risk of harsh side effects, a simple combination of natural ingredients can be applied generously to the affected area.

Activated charcoal can help minimize hormonal imbalances, remove impurities from the bloodstream, and improve circulation to optimize skin health. By consuming 1 teaspoon of activated charcoal dissolved in 1 cup of water every day, you can correct internal upsets that contribute to age spot appearance. You can also use the following recipe to create a morning salve to apply to your age spots.

TO CREATE THE AGE SPOT SALVE, USE:

1 teaspoon activated charcoal powder
1 tablespoon aloe vera
¼ cup coconut oil

Combine the ingredients and apply to the age spot–afflicted area daily. You'll see minimization of age spots in as little as 1–3 weeks. This treatment can be stored in an airtight glass container in a cool, dark area for up to 30 days, making it available for use as often as necessary.

SKIN CARE: THE BESTSELLING BEAUTY PRODUCT

The skin care industry is ever-growing and pumps out millions of products designed to fight wrinkles, blemishes, and skin abnormalities. Countless dollars are spent on these products every year, and manufacturers are well aware that consumers will risk their health on questionable ingredients that promise to deliver results. Instead of risking the health of your skin, body, and mind, opt for natural ingredients, like activated charcoal, instead.

87: PREVENTS CRACKING OF SKIN ON FEET

All the walking, sitting, and standing that you do every day at work, at home, and on the go can become exhausting to your feet. In addition to the physical toll on your feet, they may also succumb to serious skin conditions as a result of all this activity. Whether you make an effort to wear comfortable shoes as you move through your daily routine or choose to go sans shoes throughout a majority of your day, your feet can be exposed to moisture, organic elements, chemical compounds, and toxicity that can all contribute to the development of dry skin. While this may seem like a common skin issue that can be resolved with moisturizer applications, this simplistic solution may not be enough.

With the addition of activated charcoal, you can optimize the health of your skin naturally and alleviate the issues that can contribute to skin cracking, irritation, inflammation, and infection.

A simple activated charcoal foot bath can extract impurities and toxins from your feet while delivering anti-inflammatory benefits that can aid in the skin's healthy repair. The solution will also provide the feet with antibacterial, antimicrobial, and anti-fungal benefits that protect against infection. The coconut oil in this bath helps ensure that the feet remain moisturized for longer than most store-bought moisturizers can promise, leaving feet feeling naturally smooth.

TO CREATE A REJUVENATING FOOT BATH, USE:

1½ gallons warm water
1 tablespoon activated charcoal powder
½ cup coconut oil
½ cup Epsom salt

In a foot bath, combine the warm water with the rest of the ingredients and swirl to mix. Soak feet daily in the solution.

88: MAKES A NATURAL DEODORANT

Almost everyone deals with some form of body odor throughout their lifetime. There are countless products that promise to provide you with relief from the excessive sweating and smell that can result from overactive sweat glands, bacterial growth, and hormonal dysfunction, but these products may fail to relieve the body odor and can even exacerbate the underlying physical conditions that contribute to it, such as poor blood health and a seriously compromised immune system or lymphatic system. That's why using aluminum-filled, synthetic ingredient–packed deodorants and antiperspirants often causes body odor to inadvertently intensify.

With the use of an activated charcoal cleanse that can be ingested daily, the internal imbalances and issues that sometimes result in body odor can be treated effectively and quickly. In just one week, a daily teaspoon of activated charcoal can help detoxify the body and return its cells, organs, systems, and glands to their optimal functioning patterns. Consuming that dose in conjunction with a topical approach can address odor issues both internally and externally.

TO MAKE A NATURAL DEODORANT, USE:

½ cup witch hazel

1 teaspoon baking soda

½ teaspoon activated charcoal powder

Whisk the ingredients together. Move the solution to a spray bottle so it can be spritzed on areas that experience body odor, or dab on the solution using a cotton ball or towelette.

"ORGANIC" PRODUCTS FOR DEODORIZING

Many deodorants and antiperspirants contain aluminum, inorganic compounds, and synthetic additives. While some products claim to be organic, these mainstream manufactured varieties of deodorants can still contain harsh additives. Using all-natural varieties of odor-ridding cleansers and deodorizers (like activated charcoal) not only reduces body odor but also boosts health naturally too.

89: PROMOTES BONE STRENGTH AND HEALTH

There are millions of people around the globe who suffer from chronic conditions related to bone density loss. Whether the condition is due to fractures, joint pain, nervous system dysfunction, or even tooth loss, the calcium-rich deposits that make up a considerable number of usable features throughout the body can degrade over time and lead to countless painful and even life-threatening conditions. With osteoporosis, osteoarthritis, tooth loss, gingivitis, and a higher prevalence of bone damage all resulting from low calcium retention, scientists and researchers have shifted their focus from solely determining risk factors to expanding upon those risks with preventative measures that can help build, retain, and maintain calcium stores throughout the body. These natural vitamins, minerals, antioxidants, and phytochemicals that ensure the proper processes throughout the body function as intended can all contribute to the very important parts of the body that rely on calcium: the nerves, brain function, muscle mass, joint health, and the actual framework of the body (the skeletal system).

While seemingly unrelated to a bone health condition, activated charcoal can have beneficial effects on numerous cells, organs, and systems that contribute to the functions that are directly related to nutrient absorption and delivery to the sites of bone and calcium-rich stores. Through optimization of calcium absorption in the digestive system, improved blood flow for maximized delivery of calcium throughout the bloodstream, and increased capacity to store the calcium and assisting nutrients that improve calcium retention and utilization, 1 teaspoon of activated charcoal powder dissolved in 1 cup of water to be consumed daily can reduce the risk of calcium-depletion related health risks and conditions. Simply and easily, you can use activated charcoal doses to not only detoxify and prevent illnesses and health issues, but prolong the life of joints and bones!

90: ELIMINATES BACTERIA FROM THE MOUTH

While there are countless positive bacteria that help support healthy living, there are also detrimental bacteria that can quickly multiply and wreak havoc on overall health, including inside the mouth. When "bad" bacteria infiltrate the gums, teeth, and tongue, the results can be as mild as bad breath and as severe as serious disease. There are a number of products that promise to rid the mouth of bacteria, but consumers often end up with only temporary relief rather than a long-lasting defense against bacteria.

One of the most effective long-term treatments for combatting bacteria in the mouth is activated charcoal. Not only is this completely organic compound void of toxins and pathogens, it can help extract and absorb the very bacteria, viruses, and microbes that plague the mouth.

Simply combine ¼ teaspoon of activated charcoal with ¼ teaspoon of water to form a paste, and apply to a toothbrush and use it to scrub the surfaces of the mouth in order to rid the entire area of bacteria. In addition to this topical application, an ingested teaspoon of activated charcoal dissolved in 1 cup of water daily can help protect the body from bacterial infections, promote the body's natural immunity, and prevent the chronic and acute illnesses and diseases that are caused by harmful bacteria in the mouth.

BACTERIA FOR GOOD…AND BAD

With bacteria in almost every area and on every surface around us in our natural environment, it can be hard to differentiate between the good and the bad. Using activated charcoal takes the guesswork out of maintaining a healthy balance by only targeting and absorbing the bad bacteria, leaving behind the good bacteria that helps promote better overall health in your body's systems.

91: MINIMIZES VARICOSE VEINS

The veins play an important part in supporting the entire body's cells, organs, and systems. These intricate avenues of essential blood supplies provide every aspect of the body with blood, oxygen, and nutrients. When veins become compromised with blockages or get damaged by injury or illness, the result can be purple, bulbous, uncomfortable, and irritating varicose veins.

Built-up dead blood cells cause a colorful array of green, blue, red, and purple hues that track throughout the legs, ankles, and feet like road maps that lead from one coagulated area to the next. There are many creams, potions, and invasive procedures that promise to relieve varicose veins and make the veins less obvious. These approaches can be dangerous, though, and could possibly exacerbate the issue, causing more veins to become afflicted with damaging blockages.

With a combination of activated charcoal and bromelain, a topical application and an ingested application can be used to purge the veins of impurities and help alleviate unsightly varicose veins naturally. By consuming a combination of 1 teaspoon of activated charcoal dissolved in 1 cup of water and 1,000 milligrams of bromelain in supplement form daily, you can help purge the veins of the obstructive elements and dead blood cells that cause varicose veins. You can also make a salve to apply topically. Using these two applications daily, you can effectively reduce the appearance of varicose veins within a matter of weeks!

TO MAKE THE SALVE, USE:

1 teaspoon activated charcoal powder

1,000 milligrams bromelain in capsule form

1 tablespoon aloe vera

Combine all the ingredients and apply the salve directly to the site of varicose veins.

Wrap with a moist towelette or gauze and secure with a bandage or plastic wrap.

Leave on for 4 hours. Use daily.

RECOMMENDATIONS FOR USE:

This treatment can be stored in an airtight glass container in a cool, dark area for up to 30 days, making it available for use as often as necessary.

92: IMPROVES NAIL GROWTH

The rate of growth for nails varies among people, but the desire to have long, strong, beautiful nails is so widespread that manufacturers produce a multitude of products that promise perfect nails. Many of these products, whether a pill or a polish, can be packed with unhealthy ingredients that actually degrade the nails. The nails are such a thin layer of hardened protein that anything applied to them gets absorbed directly into the bloodstream, dispersing any chemicals, additives, and preservatives in nail polish and other nail treatments throughout the body. In order to prevent toxicity, infection, and inflammation, it is imperative that anyone hoping to achieve stronger, longer, healthier nails uses a natural approach.

With a diet rich in healthy fats and proteins, anyone can support the systems that promote strong hair, skin, and nail growth. In addition to a healthy diet, proper circulation is absolutely necessary to deliver essential nutrients and adequate blood supplies to the nail beds. A single teaspoon of activated charcoal dissolved in 1 cup of water consumed daily can absorb and evacuate toxicity, impurities, and obstructive elements from all parts of the body naturally. Adding a charcoal-infused nail soak can deliver moisturizing, supportive nutrients while relieving the nails and nail beds of impurities. These two applications can be used in combination to maximize the benefits to the nails, help resolve underlying issues that would obstruct healthy nail growth, and ensure that the nails grow as desired.

TO MAKE A SOAKING SOLUTION, USE:

1 teaspoon activated charcoal powder

¼ cup aloe vera

¼ cup coconut oil

Combine the ingredients in a bowl and soak the nails for 15–30 minutes.

RECOMMENDATIONS FOR USE:

This treatment can be stored in an airtight glass container in a cool, dark area for up to 30 days, making it available for use as often as necessary.

93: REDUCES APPEARANCE OF BRUISING

When you get injured, broken blood vessels can collect beneath the skin's surface at the site of the damage, causing a green, blue, or purple appearance. These broken and damaged blood cells appear discolored for between three days and three weeks on average, depending upon the severity of the damage.

If the bruise's appearance continues to worsen, spread, and become tender over time, it may be necessary to contact a physician. The spreading of damaged or dead blood cells that fail to purge from the bloodstream naturally can lead to blood clots that travel throughout the body and cause serious complications or even death.

Activated charcoal is able to help with bruising in a number of ways. With the ability to absorb and adsorb impurities in the cells and bloodstream, activated charcoal extracts the toxic substances that can impede the removal of damaged and dead blood cells. Activated charcoal also helps break down coagulated blood cells, interfering with the creation of clots and purging unhealthy elements that can interfere with healthy blood flow and circulation. A simple teaspoon of activated charcoal dissolved in 1 cup of water ingested daily can promote proper circulatory system functions and contribute to healthy circulation.

TRY USING THIS TOPICAL CHARCOAL CREAM TO TREAT BRUISING AND TENDERNESS:

1 tablespoon activated charcoal powder

1 teaspoon turmeric

¼ cup aloe vera

Combine all ingredients in an airtight glass container and apply the solution to the site of a bruise.

Wrap the area with gauze or a moist towelette and secure with a bandage or plastic wrap.

Leave the application on for 4 hours at a time.

RECOMMENDATIONS FOR USE:

This treatment can be stored in an airtight glass container in a cool, dark area for up to 30 days, making it available for use as often as necessary.

BROMELAIN FOR BRUISING

Pineapple is not only a sweet treat that can be added to smoothies, meals, and desserts but also a natural anti-inflammatory that can reduce the appearance of bruises. In addition to its immunity-boosting abundance of vitamin C, this bright fruit contains a unique phytochemical, bromelain, that helps rid the bloodstream of dead blood cells and restore health to existing blood cells.

94: REVITALIZES THE BODY WITH AN ACTIVATED CHARCOAL–BERRY LEMONADE

Whether the issue is digestion, mental clarity, energy production, or even a chronic condition (such as diabetes or obesity), activated charcoal can help the body renew its own cells, cleanse the body of impurities, and protect the cells, organs, and systems. In addition to the detoxifying benefits of activated charcoal, the vitamin C and unique phytochemicals, *limonins*, from the lemons, combined with the revitalizing vitamins, minerals, and antioxidants of the berries contribute to countless health-improving effects throughout the body. These nutrient-rich ingredients all work synergistically to improve blood quality and circulation, immune system functioning, digestion, and cell health, which support the rejuvenating processes that contribute to energy production, stamina, cognitive functioning, and cell health and vitality.

The health benefits of this drink exceed those of store-bought wellness beverages because the activated charcoal, organic fruits, and purified water all work in tandem to deliver essential nutrients while eliminating harmful elements that can plague the body with illness. Made at home and with all-natural ingredients, this beneficial beverage doesn't require preservatives, additives, or even sweeteners.

TO MAKE 8 SERVINGS OF ACTIVATED CHARCOAL–BERRY LEMONADE TONIC, USE:

7 large lemons, cleaned and sliced

1 cup raspberries

1 cup strawberries

1 tablespoon fine activated charcoal powder

2 gallons purified water

1 tablespoon mint leaves (optional)

In a large pitcher, muddle berries and lemon slices together until completely emulsified.

Add charcoal to the pitcher and stir.

Pour water over all ingredients and stir. Add mint leaves (if using).

Refrigerate for 8 hours to allow all ingredients to combine thoroughly, stirring occasionally.

RECOMMENDATIONS FOR USE:

Consume 8 ounces every 4 hours.

95: REMOVES TOXINS WITH A SPIRULINA AND CHARCOAL GREEN SMOOTHIE

Green smoothies can be challenging to add to your diet...especially if greens haven't been a welcome staple in your everyday meals. Introducing a healthy dose of pH-balancing spinach and kale to cleanse the colon and support the immune system, this simple smoothie not only tastes great and can be made quickly and easily, but it also delivers countless benefits to the body and mind. In addition to nutritional support, the smoothie has the added cleansing benefit of activated charcoal that helps the body purge toxins and impurities naturally. The recipe combines fibrous greens, activated charcoal powder, and protein-rich spirulina for a simple and easy drink that tastes great and helps support the natural functioning of the body.

In a large blender, combine all ingredients.

Blend on high until all ingredients are emulsified and thoroughly combined.

Consume immediately, reserving any remaining smoothie in an airtight container in the refrigerator for up to 2 days.

SPIRULINA'S AMAZING ABILITIES TO PROVIDE PROTEIN

While vegetarianism is growing popular, the concern of inadequate protein intake is commonly discussed among medical and natural health professionals. However, with the addition of spirulina to the daily diet, the body's natural requirements for protein are met in such a manner that requires little digestive effort, boosts immune system functioning, and provides astounding amounts of essential nutrients.

TO MAKE 2 SERVINGS OF THE SPIRULINA AND CHARCOAL GREEN SMOOTHIE, USE:

4 cups purified water

1 cup spinach

½ cup kale

1 tablespoon spirulina powder

1 tablespoon activated charcoal powder

1 medium apple, cored

96: RESTORES HEALTH WITH A GINGER AND CHARCOAL–INFUSED GREEN TEA

In this delightful recipe, three amazing ingredients combine to create a refreshing tonic that not only restores health and rejuvenates the mind but also satisfies the taste buds and calms cravings. Spicy gingerroot invigorates the metabolic system for optimized circulation, nutrient processing, and digestion relief, enabling the absorption of every phytochemical and proactive antioxidant that green tea provides. The activated charcoal in this green tea tonic helps rid the body of undesirable elements, such as toxins, impurities, and pathogens, that regularly interfere with the body's natural processing. Cleansing the mind and body of harmful elements that interfere with every process imaginable, this simple green tea recipe can be sipped in place of coffee, as a snack throughout the day, or alongside any meal.

TO MAKE 8 CUPS OF THIS TEA, USE:

8 cups purified water
1" piece gingerroot, peeled and sliced
4 organic green tea bags
1 tablespoon activated charcoal powder

In a large pot, boil water. Remove from heat.

Add sliced gingerroot, green tea bags, and activated charcoal.

Stir ingredients to combine thoroughly, cover, and allow to steep for 8 hours.

Refrigerate remaining tea for up to 4 days.

GINGER FOR...EVERYTHING

With potent antioxidants and abundant nutrients, as well as its ability to fight bacteria, viruses, fungi, and microbes, ginger is not just your everyday digestive upset cure. This pH-balancing root can improve blood health, brain functioning, circulation, digestion, and immunity. Combined with activated charcoal, ginger is the perfect ingredient to combat a variety of health issues.

97: CALMS CRAVINGS WITH CHARCOAL-SESAME CRACKERS

For the perfect crunchy snack, charcoal may not seem all that appetizing, but this surprisingly delicious combination of ingredients comes together to create crisp, airy crackers that are perfect as a snack, appetizer, or accompaniment for your favorite dip. Aiding in the removal of impurities from the bloodstream while improving the body's intake of essential nutrients, the addition of activated charcoal makes these delightful crackers both nutrient-rich and nutrient-absorbing. This tasty recipe makes for a satisfying snack that calms cravings and delivers everything the body and mind needs.

TO MAKE 4 SERVINGS OF CRACKERS, USE:

1 cup almond flour

3 tablespoons sesame seeds

1 teaspoon activated charcoal powder

¼ teaspoon salt

⅛ teaspoon cayenne pepper (optional)

1 large egg

Preheat oven to 350°F. Prepare a baking sheet with cooking spray or parchment paper.

Combine all ingredients and whisk or stir to mix thoroughly. Pour onto prepared baking sheet.

Bake 15–20 minutes or until golden brown.

Remove and allow to cool before cutting into thin or thick slices, depending on preference.

CAYENNE'S SPECIAL EFFECTS ON METABOLISM

Cayenne isn't just a fabulous ingredient that can spice up your favorite dishes. This delicious addition also fires up metabolic processes and invigorates the body and mind. With natural thermogenic effects that heat up the body, almost every aspect of the body's processes, from circulation to metabolism, benefit. The astounding result is an enhanced metabolism, more efficient brain, faster fat loss, and improved energy.

98: SOOTHES YOUR BODY WITH A CHARCOAL AND STRAWBERRY SORBET

On a hot afternoon, or even in the middle of the night, a sweet strawberry sorbet can soothe the body and soul. Vibrant strawberries combine with invigorating mint leaves and purifying activated charcoal for a combination of ingredients that not only refreshes the body but also helps reinvigorate the cells, organs, and systems to their optimal state. Once the body is free of toxins, it can resume its normal processing, absorption, and distribution of nutrients to support all aspects of healthy living. With every bite of this delicious, nutritious sorbet, the body, mind, and taste buds are provided with all that they need.

TO MAKE 4 SERVINGS OF SORBET, USE:

4 cups green tea, chilled

4 cups strawberries, tops removed

¼ cup mint leaves

1 teaspoon activated charcoal powder

In a large blender, combine all ingredients and blend on high until everything is macerated and thoroughly combined.

In a 13" x 9" glass dish, pour in mixture and spread evenly.

Cover the dish with plastic wrap or aluminum foil and place in the freezer for 8–12 hours.

Scrape the sorbet to create an airy, shaved ice consistency and transfer to 4 bowls.

STRAWBERRIES AND VITAMIN C

While most people associate oranges and citrus fruits with vitamin C, strawberries actually provide far more of this immunity-boosting essential than any fruity alternative. With the added benefit of anthocyanins that act as free radical–combatting protectants, strawberries are a sweet treat that add flavor and healthy essential nutrients to any meal or snack.

99: DECONTAMINATES WITH CHARCOAL–DARK CHOCOLATE BROWNIES

This simple recipe provides plentiful nutrients that not only satisfy the body's needs but also satisfy the taste buds. Nourishing the cells, organs, and systems, the activated charcoal combines with vitamins, minerals, proteins, carbohydrates, and healthy fats to create a delicious and nutritious alternative to the average everyday brownie. Replacing the processed ingredients of regular brownies with healthy alternatives, these sweet treats taste great and provide the body with guilt-free nourishment that flushes out impurities and promotes healthy functioning.

TO MAKE 16 BROWNIES, USE:

½ cup unsalted butter

1 cup sugar

2 large eggs

1 teaspoon vanilla extract

⅓ cup unsweetened cocoa powder

½ cup flour

¼ teaspoon baking powder

1 teaspoon activated charcoal powder

Preheat oven to 350°F. Prepare a 13" x 9" baking dish with nonstick cooking spray.

In a large bowl, combine all ingredients and mix thoroughly.

Pour ingredients into the dish and use a spoon to even the mixture out to the same thickness.

Bake 25 minutes or until a fork inserted in the center comes out clean.

Cool, cut into 16 equal pieces, and serve.

DARK CHOCOLATE'S ABUNDANT ANTIOXIDANTS

With the rich nutrients of dark chocolate contributing to many of the natural processes in the body, its added benefit of plentiful antioxidants is a welcome bonus for anyone hoping to achieve optimal health. Infusing the daily diet with phytochemicals, antioxidants, and free radical–combatting compounds, a simple serving of dark chocolate is good for the body and mind.

100: ELIMINATES TOXINS WITH CARAMEL-CHOCOLATE-CHARCOAL MACAROONS

There are a number of ways to transform a conventional confectionary treat into a healthy, satisfying snack that can be enjoyed without any guilt. Activated charcoal can be included in many recipes, but one of the tastiest and most effective at calming cravings is this caramel-chocolate-charcoal macaroon recipe. It not only satisfies cravings but also supplies essential nutrition to the cells, organs, and systems. The activated charcoal in this recipe is undetectable in taste, but it helps purge the body of toxicity and pathogens, recalibrating the processes that contribute to overall body health—all while being enveloped in a delicious puffy cloud of coconut and chocolate. You can enjoy these delicious and nutritious bites of goodness any time to restore energy, rejuvenate the mind, and revive the body naturally!

¾ cup sugar

1 teaspoon activated charcoal powder

¼ cup water

2 large egg whites

1½ cups almond flour

1 cup unsweetened coconut flakes

1 cup powdered sugar

¼ cup unsweetened cocoa powder

1 tablespoon melted salted caramel candy blocks or squares, melted

Preheat oven to 350°F and prepare a large baking sheet with nonstick spray.

Combine all ingredients in a high-speed mixer and blend on high speed until thoroughly combined and frothy.

Spoon mixture in tablespoon-sized servings onto baking sheet.

Bake 10–15 minutes or until golden brown.

Remove from baking sheet and allow to cool before serving.

Store in an airtight container for up to 4 days.

CHARCOAL'S CONTRIBUTION TO DIABETES

When a patient is diagnosed with diabetes or any other metabolic condition, rigid dietary restrictions can wreak havoc on daily meal planning. With activated charcoal aiding in the natural hormonal processes that govern metabolic functions, dietary restrictions can be gradually eased, allowing for sweet treats like these delicious macaroons.

INDEX

ABOUT THE AUTHOR

Britt Brandon is a Certified Personal Trainer and Certified Fitness Nutrition Specialist (certified by the International Sports Sciences Association, ISSA) and Health Coach (certified by the American Council on Exercise, ACE) who has enjoyed writing books that focus on clean eating, fitness, and unique health promoting ingredients such as apple cider vinegar, coconut oil, and aloe vera for Adams Media. In her time with Adams, she has published eleven books including *The Everything® Green Smoothies Book*, *The Everything® Eating Clean Cookbook*, *What Color Is Your Smoothie?*, *The Everything® Eating Clean Cookbook for Vegetarians*, *The Everything® Healthy Green Drinks Book*, and *The Everything® Guide to Pregnancy Nutrition & Health*. As a competitive athlete, trainer, mom of three small children, and fitness and nutrition blogger on her own website (UltimateFitMom.com), she is well versed in the holistic approaches to keeping oneself in top performing condition.